BREAKING THROUGH THE PAIN BARRIER

The extraordinary life
of
Dr Michael J. Cousins

GABRIELLA KELLY-DAVIES

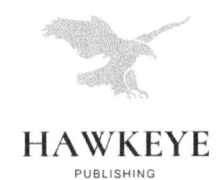

First published in Australia in 2021 by Hawkeye Publishing.

Copyright © Gabriella Kelly-Davies.

Cover Design by Ngaire McLoughlin.
This cover has been designed using resources from Flaticon.com. Quill Drawing A Line Icon made by Freepik. Book Icon made by srip.

Back Cover Portrait of Michael J. Cousins by artist Peter Smeeth, 2018. Portrait resides at Australian & New Zealand College of Anaesthetists, Melbourne.
Author's Photograph by Simona Janek.

All rights reserved. No part of this book may be reproduced, stored in a retrieval system, or transmitted, in any form or by any means, without the prior permission in writing of the publisher, nor be otherwise circulated in any form of binding or cover other than that in which it is published and without a similar condition including this condition being imposed on the subsequent purchaser.

ISBN 978-0-6450844-3-6

www.hawkeyepublishing.com.au
www.hawkeyebooks.com.au

Praise for Breaking Through the Pain Barrier

'I am enthralled and can't put the book down. The fascinating story of the man who brought pain medicine to Australia and devoted his life to the pursuit of pain relief,' **John D. Loeser M.D.,** *Pain Medicine Pioneer.*

'Sometimes the difference between the good and the great is only a higher level of vision and sheer single-minded determination… a remarkable life,' **Dr Marc A. Russo,** *Pain Medicine Specialist.*

'I always find it interesting to read of a subject's origins and see how those influenced the outcome of their life. Dr Cousins' father's legacy included a high level of values and moral responsibility, and various members of his family were change agents, compelled to right wrongs. The author has done an exceptional job of documenting important history within the frame of an interesting story,' **Cate Sawyer,** *Author.*

'This is a profoundly moving book celebrating the life and legacy of a remarkable man. As his patient and biographer, Gabriella overlooks nothing as she records Michael Cousins' ground-breaking achievements and life-long commitment to improving the treatment of pain. Gabriella reveals the victories and frustrations of Michael's medical career, as well as his great human qualities: a kind and caring physician, a loyal friend and devoted family man. This is a book to bring joy to any reader: a fellow physician or simply a fellow human being,' **Lesley Brydon AM,** *Founding CEO, Painaustralia.*

'Professor Cousins is a dedicated researcher and clinician who is committed to achieving lasting change in the way that Australia and many other countries around the world address chronic pain. I commend this book to those with an interest in making a difference in the lives of those affected by complex health and other challenges,' **Air Chief Marshal Sir Angus Houston,** *Painaustralia Patron.*

'*Breaking through the Pain Barrier* by Gabriella Kelly-Davies is a worthy tribute to Professor Michael Cousins. So many patients have benefited from the work Prof Cousins has done to improve the care of pain patients, from his holistic approach to pain and focus on brain re-training, pacing and neuroscience. It's an engaging book, showing the reader the clinician, researcher and Prof Cousins' family life as well. It offers hope to patients too, that pain can be better managed through access to holistic pain clinics and services,' **Sophie Scott,** *Journalist, Broadcaster, Author & Pain Champion.*

'Michael Cousins is a rare person whose vision for pain management is matched by his intellect and compassion. Michael's work has made a difference to the lives of not only Australians but those living with pain conditions everywhere,' **Robert Regan,** *Former Chair, Painaustralia, Group General Counsel and Company Secretary, Downer Group.*

'A meticulous, inspiring study of one extraordinary life. The author's compelling and passionate account shows how medicine can be transformed by the power of one individual. This work of integrity and compassion offers us some much-needed hope,' **Lee Kofman,** *Author of Imperfect.*

'The proper management of pain remains, after all, the most important obligation, the main objective and the crowning achievement of every physician,'

John J. Bonica, The Management of Pain, 1953.

CONTENTS

Dedication

Foreword by Dr Marc A. Russo   iii

Prologue   v

1	Learning About Pain	1
2	Montreal	13
3	Stanford	28
4	The Tug of Home	37
5	Nurturing a Fledgling	43
6	The Race to Advance Epidural Pain Relief	53
7	The Power of Relationships	63
8	Playing on the World Stage	73
9	Starting Over	85
10	Advancing Pain Research	93
11	Chronic Pain: Michael's patients share their stories	97
12	The Troubling Transition	110
13	Birth of the Pain Management Research Institute	121
14	The 2000s	130
15	New Frontiers	148

16	Pain Gets a Seat at the Table	163
17	Closing a Chapter	173
	Epilogue	189
	Afterword by Carol Bennett	191
	Notes	193
	Acknowledgements	194
	About the Author	195
	Bibliography	196

DEDICATION

To the 1 in 5 people who live with chronic pain.

FOREWORD

BIOGRAPHIES of doctors often come in two well-worn formats. Either they appear as dry dusty tomes of chronological events and scientific minutiae of indecipherable relevance to the average reader, or they appear as breathy hagiographies where with seeming omnipotence the biographical subject breezes through their life with preternatural ability. This book is neither.

It occupies a small niche of biographies where the reader gets to 'look under the hood' at not only what was accomplished but how it was attained and the very human feelings of failure, success and doubt as travails were undertaken. This book will give you not only a very real sense of the man who is MJC and what drives him, but also how random twists of events and doses of good luck can influence outcomes.

To some extent and certainly viewing from afar, I assumed MJC achieved everything he turned his hand to with consummate ease. Little did I realise in my naiveté the extent of the 'grunt work' necessary to stoke the engine of change. Sometimes the difference between the good and the great is only a higher level of vision and sheer single-minded determination.

Although the author has significant experience of writing biographies, here she has tackled a task that is tricky and perspective challenging. For Gabriella not only knew her subject, but was a patient of his, as she details in the book. This presents a unique challenge to any biographer to present an unadorned truth to their subject—especially in those still living—and is one she has executed here with aplomb.

This biography will captivate several types of readers. Obviously, it will appeal to the pain treatment community—and should certainly feature in the library of every pain clinic in the southern and northern hemispheres. People suffering from persistent pain who wish to understand how their medical system has come into being will also appreciate it. The book will interest—and have some profound insights for—anyone interested in how to create change within institutions, medical or otherwise. It will also intrigue those curious about reaching the heights of human endeavour. There are plenty of books written about climbers of the tallest mountains on earth, but there is also much to learn from studying those who have climbed mountains of inertia and changed societal and cultural responses to how our own bodies are treated by fellow humans.

I have a much deeper appreciation of MJC from this book—and discovered a remarkably shared dislike of clothes shopping! To me, this biography shows the true time value of persistence and how, almost like the power of compound interest, the power of persistence can accumulate over time and create wonderful things. Without biographies like this, charting the innermost workings of a career, scholars two hundred years from now would have only a few plaques and awards to define a very human human being. Gabriella Kelly-Davies has done much, much more than that. She has done justice to her subject and let us inside his remarkable life.

Dr Marc A. Russo
Specialist Pain Medicine Physician, Newcastle, Australia.

PROLOGUE

TWO little boys stand transfixed in front of a roaring bonfire in their backyard. Earlier in the day, they helped their dad mow the lawn and burn the clippings in the incinerator; then they watered the garden with the dark green hose. Afterwards, they ran in circles, giggling, while their mother tied red balloons to the Hills Hoist.

It is cracker night in 1964 and like thousands of kids across New South Wales, the brothers squeal with delight every time their father stands a skyrocket in an empty milk bottle and lights the fuse. They watch in awe as it blasts into the air, spraying a rainbow of colours high above their heads. Once the thrill of the skyrocket wears off their dad lights a double bunger that makes an ear-splitting racket when it explodes.

The boys' mother places platters of hot party pies and sausage rolls on the fold-up picnic table near the shed and pours tomato sauce into a round dish. She pulls the caps from two small bottles of Coca-Cola. The children toss throwdowns onto the path, watching them explode with a boom and bright sparks.

'Dinner's ready,' the mother calls.

'Oh, *Mum*. One more throwdown?'

'Yes, just one more, then wash your—.' A sudden gust of wind blows flames from the bonfire towards the children, engulfing them. The mother drops a glass jug of water. She runs across to her sons. So does their father.

They roll their children on the damp grass to put out the flames.

'Grab the car keys,' the father yells. 'We'll drive them to the hospital. It'll be quicker than waiting for an ambulance.'

The mother runs into the house and fetches the keys. She also rings St George Hospital to tell them her sons are on their way.

The father drives. The boys' mother sits in the back seat trying to console her sons, and before the car stops at Emergency, she flings open the rear door. She tries to carry one boy, but he brushes her away. The boys limp up the path, crying, 'Save me. Save me.'

A young man with dark hair runs towards them. He wears a white coat and a stethoscope swings from his neck. As he gets closer to the children, he realises they are the two burned boys he was waiting for in the ambulance bay.

This young man is twenty-five-year-old Dr Michael Cousins. He had finished medical school twelve months earlier and is now a resident medical officer at St George Hospital in southern Sydney. At this stage of his career, he doesn't know which medical speciality to pursue and often worries that he might never find an area of medicine that is right for him.

Michael notes the skin on the boys' faces is black and the skin on their heads, torso, arms and legs looks completely burned off. The boys sob, and their blackened hair stands on end, making it look fuzzy.

Once the boys are inside the emergency department, Michael gently inserts needles into the backs of their burned hands. The needles are attached to drips. Their hands balloon and he is glad he got the cannulas in on time—any later, and the swelling would have prevented it. Michael runs tiny doses of morphine through the drips, then places oxygen masks over the boys' scorched faces. But the morphine doesn't work. The children's screams continue.

For the next forty-eight hours, Michael and the hospital's medical and nursing team keep a vigil by the boys' bedsides. They save the children's lives but struggle to ease their suffering.

That weekend Michael Cousins made a decision that would define his future—he committed his life to reducing suffering by improving the treatment of pain.

1

LEARNING ABOUT PAIN

THE pain the two burned boys endured haunted Michael. He felt out of his depth trying to reduce their suffering and realised his medical training had not equipped him to control such severe pain. 'I guess it impressed on me the need to have something a lot better,' he recalls. He was not sure how to specialise in pain, but asked the senior doctors at his hospital if they knew. Pain was such a new field of medicine that few people knew about it. A few of them suggested he train as an anaesthetist because in the 1960s it was anaesthetists who treated patients with excruciating pain. 'It didn't take me long to realise that to find the right spot for me in medicine, I needed to get onto the road of anaesthesia training.'

In January 1965, six months after treating the burned boys, Michael joined Royal North Shore Hospital in Sydney as an anaesthesia registrar. He felt 'at home' at the hospital because he often bumped into his mother Marjorie in the lift or corridors—she worked there as a volunteer. During medical school, Michael too had worked at the hospital, but as a porter in the chest surgery ward. As a fourteen-year-old, he had been a patient at Royal North Shore Hospital after he broke his nose playing rugby and required surgery. This experience lit the fire to study medicine, although an earlier exposure to medicine may have also been pivotal in his career choice. When Michael was ten years old, his next-door neighbour gave him a copy of the surgeon Dr John Hilton's classic book *Rest and Pain*.[1] It was a series of lectures on anatomy and pain that John Hilton delivered between 1860 and 1862. Hilton was a member of the Royal College of Surgeons in England, and he expressed novel ideas about how acute pain could interfere with, or help, people recovering from surgery. 'I was fascinated by that book,' Michael said. 'It was one of the most insightful books of the nineteenth century. I read it many times.'[2] Michael has no idea why his neighbour gave him the book and to this day remains intrigued that he was introduced to pain as a topic at such a young age.

On his first day as a registrar, Michael treated several patients in the emergency department – a small room with two beds separated by short calico curtains. One patient was a tall, muscular man in his thirties. The man walked stiffly and his shoulders sagged.

'I've had pain in my back for two years,' the man said, grimacing. 'It's so bad it keeps me awake at night.'

Michael asked how it had started. The man first felt it as he bent over to pick up a load of bricks on a building site. He heard a loud crack; then a sharp pain shot through his lower back. The man lifted his shirt and pointed to an area above his right buttock. 'It's in here, Doc. It's deep down. An electric shock runs down my right leg.' Michael asked what made the pain worse and the man told him that lifting heavy objects hurt, especially bending down to pick up his kids. He said he couldn't work as a labourer anymore because it flared up the pain too much.

At that stage, Michael was not sure how to help the man, but he was determined to find a way. Every time he had a spare minute, he read textbooks and spoke with professors at the hospital. As the months passed by, Michael met many patients like the man he saw on his first day. He worried about them. Patient after patient told him how their GP had sent them to a specialist who referred them to another specialist. But none of the doctors could reduce their pain.

Michael empathised with his patients because he had suffered agonising abdominal cramps since childhood. As a young boy, they sometimes hit him when he was walking to school. The pain was so bad he crumpled into the gutter waiting for it to ease. The problem continued during his teenage years and still affected him as an adult. He too had seen specialist after specialist, but no-one could offer him any relief. Other than the abdominal pain, Michael had been a robust child and a talented athlete. Every night, he had joined his childhood friends Ray Chapman and Fergus Munro for athletic training in Ray's backyard. Their regimen included a series of strenuous callisthenics, weight training, throwing shot-puts and sprints. Michael was so determined to succeed he diligently saved his pocket money towards buying handmade running shoes with spikes from a specialist shoemaker in Sydney. He had maintained a strict diet, avoiding any food that wouldn't enhance his performance—his only exception was his mother's irresistible, ultra-sweet caramel tart. So his cramps remained a mystery to everyone concerned.

Every night after work at Royal North Shore Hospital, Michael raced home to read journal articles about pain. He lived with his parents, Marjorie and Hedley Cousins, and brother Geoff on Sydney's upper North Shore because he was saving to buy a flat. Geoff was three years younger than Michael and the two brothers shared a love of tennis, rugby and athletics. Michael and Geoff had a much older brother and sister from Hedley's first marriage—when Michael was born in 1939, Keith was fourteen and Pam eleven. Tragically, their mother, Lavinia, died of tuberculosis when they were children.

Marjorie was a loving mother, but she was the controlling influence and disciplinarian in her home. Tall and slim, with short brown hair, she enjoyed playing golf and was an accomplished tennis player. Also active in the community, Marjorie was known locally as a 'change agent', stepping in whenever she thought something was wrong. This tendency to identify an issue, take action and bring about change was a feature of Michael's extended family and it was deeply ingrained in him from a young age.

A 'gentlemanly' figure, Hedley Leunig Cousins was tall and wore glasses. Distinguished looking, he spoke with his hands, enthusiastically gesturing during his conversations. He loved smoking his pipe and family folklore suggests he smoked it upside down in the shower. Personable and kind, Hedley wasn't religious and instead lived by a high moral code he would instil in Michael. He didn't hold firm political beliefs or strong opinions on social issues, which is surprising given the paths his three sons followed. Hedley was a senior account manager at the advertising agency, Jackson Wayne, and quickly climbed the corporate ladder because of his exceptional communication skills. He would later head the company.

Once pain management became his passion, Michael spent his evenings buried in books. Every night immediately after dinner with his parents and Geoff, he headed to the makeshift study he had created under his family's bungalow. Bookshelves filled with dog-eared textbooks lined the walls, and white index cards covered in tiny writing and drawings littered his desk. Sitting at the oak desk late into the night, he searched for clues on how to reduce his patients' pain. One night he read that an authoritative textbook had been written on pain. *I must find it*, he thought, impatient to read the book he hoped would help him reduce his patients' pain. He scribbled the book's details in a notebook then placed it in his battered leather briefcase.

At the crack of dawn the following Saturday Michael jolted awake, even though his last shift for the week had ended only a few hours earlier. After a breakfast of wheatgerm and molasses—'terrible stuff' that sporting coaches touted as increasing athletic performance—he drove to Sydney University. He stood at the library's locked door, checking his watch every few minutes. It was cold standing outside the old sandstone building, so he stamped his feet and rubbed his hands to warm up.

On the dot of nine o'clock, a small woman with short grey hair opened the glass doors. Michael smelled the familiar musty odour that brought back memories of spending long hours studying in the library. He headed straight to the catalogue; a series of wooden drawers filled with white index cards then looked up 'B'. 'Yes! He's here,' Michael gasped, barely able to contain his excitement. He had found Professor John J. Bonica's hefty textbook from 1953 *The Management of Pain*[3] – the only book that discussed everything known about pain and its treatment. Michael made a beeline for the shelf that held the key to his future, hurriedly scanning the call numbers. His heart pounded against his chest wall as he glimpsed the bulky tome. He pulled it from the shelf and carried it to a desk. At the same time as he pulled out a chair, he opened the book and tried to read it. He checked the contents page, opened it to the right section, ran his finger down each page, line by line.

Michael read that John Bonica, an anaesthetist, launched a pioneering pain centre in America in the 1940s and that one way he treated his patients' pain was by injecting local anaesthetic onto a nerve to numb it. This technique is a nerve block, and Michael decided to try it on some of his patients who had endured years of unrelenting pain.

He also learned that ideas of the seventeenth-century philosopher, René Descartes, still influenced pain treatments in the 1960s. Descartes believed that pain signals travel from injured tissues in the body to a pain centre in the brain. This 'hardwired' concept of pain is like a telephone cable system with electrical impulses running from the surface of the skin to the spinal cord and then to the brain where a bell rings when the pain arrives.[4] It surprised Michael that knowledge about pain had progressed little during the previous three centuries, and he wondered how Descartes' theory applied to his patients' suffering from persistent pain. He resolved to find out.

John Bonica's textbook was in the reference section and not free to borrow, but Michael planned to spend the weekend in the library studying it. It was like a second home to him because he had studied medicine at Sydney University for six years from 1958; he often revised his lecture notes in the library before exams. A conscientious student, he was often afraid he would be among the two-thirds of students who failed each year. 'I worried that I hadn't done enough. If I failed the exam at the end of the year—out.' Still, he enjoyed socialising and was 'distracted by the nurses'. He was notorious for poking his head through the open windows of his friends' bedrooms in the middle of the night and saying, 'Get up! There's a terrific party on!'

Most days during his first months as a registrar, Michael woke up energised, despite often working thirty-six-hour shifts. These marathons involved arriving at the hospital at seven o'clock in the morning, treating patients until seven o'clock in the evening, then doing the night shift, followed by another full day of work. Along the way, he would snatch an hour or two of sleep at the hospital if he could, but this was not always possible. At his core, he was bone-tired, and his clothes reeked of anaesthetic gas from spending so many hours in the poorly ventilated operating theatres. But his passion for learning more about pain drove him. He worried that so many of his patients complained about their pain and longed to offer them more relief than was available. His relentless search for clues continued, despite the toll it took on him.

Michael often sedated patients who were having surgery on their blood vessels for problems such as varicose veins. He worked with the hospital's head surgeon, Professor Tom Reeve, an 'old school professor and a gentleman,' according to Michael.

One day after an operation Reeve took Michael aside. 'I'm disappointed when some of my patients wake up from surgery shivering and in pain,' Reeve said in his warm, gentle voice. Michael nodded as he knew that shivering caused the arteries and veins to narrow. If this happened after surgery, it could stop blood flowing into the fresh blood vessel graft, and the graft could die. Reeve asked Michael if he had learned about the problem at medical school. Michael shook his head but said he would research it.

During the following week, Michael stayed up late searching medical journals for answers, and he found articles by McGill University's Professor Philip Bromage, the doyen of regional anaesthesia.[i] Bromage described how he had injected local anaesthetic into the epidural space—the space surrounding the outer membrane of the spinal cord—to relieve pain after patients had crushed their chests in an accident. This procedure reduced the discomfort, enabling patients to cough, remove any secretions from their lungs, and recover more quickly. Michael wondered if an epidural anaesthetic might reduce shivering and pain after blood vessel surgery.

The next day he hurried to the hospital and scouted around for Professor Reeve. When he found him, he said, 'I've been thinking about the shivering problem. I thought that running local anaesthetic into the epidural space after the operation might help. It could continue the effects of the epidural anaesthetic given during surgery.'

Reeve thought it an unorthodox idea, but was keen to test it. When they did, they noticed the number of patients who shivered after their operation dropped. And more of Reeve's blood vessel grafts survived. This result intrigued Michael. He started to dream up ideas for research projects that might help him discover why the postoperative epidural anaesthesia had reduced shivering.

Around the same time, Michael met Michele Old at a Christmas party. Michele had just finished an arts degree at Sydney University and was a member of the university's ski team. Petite, with golden blonde hair and translucent blue eyes, she worked as a research assistant at Sydney University's law school. Michele took one look at Michael's warm hazel eyes and friendly smile and instinctively knew they would marry. Michael felt the same. 'It felt as if we'd known each other all our lives. It was most peculiar, as it happened in an instant.' Michael drove Michele home and invited her to dinner. But to his dismay, he had to wait six anxious days for his date because Michele was busy with pre-Christmas festivities.

Two weeks after meeting Michele, Michael asked her to marry him. To his delight, she accepted. Down at Palm Beach two weeks later at Michele's parents' home, Michael seized the moment, asking Michele's father, Trenham, for permission to marry his daughter.

Trenham looked startled. 'You haven't known each other very long, have you?' he asked, accidently pouring his wife, Poppy, a glass of whiskey AND brandy. Still, he agreed to his future son-in-law's request.

Michael agrees that asking Michele to marry him after only two weeks of knowing her was the rashest decision of his life and out of character for him. He usually thinks carefully about decisions, agonising over the pros and cons. But in the case of marrying Michele, he insists it wasn't ever a decision because he knew she was the 'right one' from the moment he met her.

Michael and Michele became engaged, but they waited until the end of March 1967 to announce it because Michael was determined to pass the first part of the anaesthesia fellowship exam, and he didn't want any distractions to disturb his study schedule. For several long weeks he studied 'flat out' whenever he wasn't working at the hospital. Immediately after the exam, and one week before Marjorie and Hedley Cousins were due to leave for a seven-month trip overseas, the young couple held an engagement party at Michele's home and another at Michael's place.

For the next seven months, while waiting for Michael's parents to return, the duo dated whenever Michael had a break from work and study. But he yearned to spend more time with Michele and missed her when they were apart. On the nights they went out together, he picked her up in the little cream Morris 1100 he had purchased while a resident medical officer at St George Hospital. In 1958, shortly before starting medical school, he bought a green 1911 Chrysler that cost £25. Unfortunately, it 'chewed petrol' and it was a bit greasy, but it had a fifth seat like a London taxi that folded out from the boot. While a student he felt proud of his car, but once he graduated, realised he needed 'to do a lot better'. Once he had saved enough, he purchased the Morris, even though it cost more than he felt he could afford. Michael and Michele enjoyed movies and parties, and they loved going to Sydney Symphony Orchestra concerts in Sydney Town Hall. They also skied during winter—Michele relished the perilous black runs. Michael was also game although he preferred to 'play it safe' on less risky slopes.

Ten days after Hedley and Marjorie Cousins arrived home—on 27 October 1967—Michael and Michele married at St Martins Anglican Church in Killara. They had both been christened and confirmed there. Michele was twenty-three and Michael twenty-eight. Michael caught his breath and felt his eyes fill with tears as he watched Michele enter the large wooden front door then gracefully walk up the aisle. She wore a white double silk organza dress, with three-quarter length sleeves and a modest scoop neck. Her veil cascaded over her slim shoulders and the tulle train, which her sister Rosemary guided along the floor, streamed behind her. She held a bouquet made from white Stephanotis and Lily of the Valley. Michael wore black tails, a white bowtie and white gloves. His brother, Geoff, was his best man and Michele's brother, Rick, was a groomsman.

The next day the newlyweds flew to Noumea for their honeymoon.

They loved the blue lagoons and crystal-clear waters of the island, and they spent blissful days swimming, snorkelling and sailing. They had planned to visit Fiji and then go on to New Zealand, but when they reached Fiji, Michael said, 'What are we doing? Why don't we just stop here?' So they holidayed in Fiji for two weeks rather than heading to New Zealand. They luxuriated, relaxing under the tall palm trees, reading novels and chatting. It was the most time they had spent together since meeting the year before.

When Michael and Michele returned from their honeymoon, they moved into Granny Cousins' furnished unit in Werona Avenue, Gordon. To their delight, Michael's paternal grandmother, May, offered it to them at half the standard rent. It was a great relief, enabling the couple to live on Michael's salary and save Michele's small income. The flat was next to tennis courts and across the road from Gordon railway station, so Michele travelled to the law school by train every day. Michael drove his old Morris the twenty minutes it took to get to the hospital. Occasionally it broke down, so he would jog home to grab Michele's Volkswagen Beetle to drive to work, fretting he would arrive late for ward rounds.

On weekends the newlyweds stayed at Poppy and Trenham's holiday house at Palm Beach so Michael could combine studying for the second part of the anaesthesia fellowship exam with walking, sprinting and bodysurfing. He revelled in feeling the salty summer breeze on his face. The couple had little time for parties and entertaining because Michael was so busy working and studying, but Michele encouraged him to study in bed and she snuggled up next to him reading novels. 'I knew what I was signing up for in marrying a doctor,' she recalls.[5]

During 1968, a well-known English anaesthetist, Professor Gordon Robson, toured Australia and one afternoon gave a lecture at Royal North Shore Hospital. About twenty doctors and nurses sat in the brightly lit meeting room listening to Robson speak about his anaesthesia research at McGill University in Montreal. The doctors and nurses ate ham, cheese and tomato sandwiches and sipped lukewarm cups of tea. Every so often they checked their watches or beeping pagers. Telephones rang in the background, and ceiling fans whirred overhead.

Michael was one of the doctors in the room. He had arrived late because the last operation of the morning took longer than expected. Still dressed in the green surgical gown he wore in the operating theatre, he worried he had missed Robson's opening remarks. As he sat down in the front row, he opened his notebook to a clean page and tuned in to what the professor was saying.

While Robson explained his latest research project, Michael sat transfixed, intent on learning everything he could from the eminent professor. Unlike the others, he feverishly scribbled notes on a writing pad. His untouched sandwich sat on the chair beside him.

At the end of the lecture, Michael jumped up before the applause ended. He introduced himself to Robson, and they chatted about the professor's research. Michael asked him whether he worked with Philip Bromage.

'Would you like to work with Professor Bromage?' Robson said with an amused look on his face.

Michael nodded, almost in disbelief, and asked what he needed to do to work at McGill.

'Leave it with me,' Robson said, before turning to speak with one of Michael's colleagues.

Months passed. Then one day in 1968 Michael found a letter waiting for him at the hospital. The envelope was pillar-box red.

'I wonder who it's from?' he thought, as he sliced it open with a pen. It had a Canadian postmark.

'It's a letter from Gordon Robson!' he gasped.

He read the letter. 'It's all fixed. I've spoken to Philip Bromage. He'd love to have you at McGill, so go to it.' He couldn't wait to get home to tell Michele, but he had a busy afternoon in the operating theatre to get through first.

That night after dinner Michael stayed up late writing a letter to Sydney University. He asked the postgraduate foundation for a scholarship so he and Michele could travel to Montreal to research epidural pain relief with Philip Bromage.

In the letter, Michael laid out his idea for a research study that would involve placing tiny electrodes in the epidural space to create an electric current that might block pain signals travelling to the brain. This concept was novel, but Michael thought it might have a similar effect to injecting local anaesthetic into the epidural space—but without the complications of local anaesthesia such as loss of feeling and movement in the legs.

Early the next morning, Michael dropped his application into the hospital's mailbox. Then he hurried to a meeting with the hospital's senior managers. A few months earlier, his colleagues had elected him to chair the 'House Committee', a group of staff who lobbied the hospital's administrators to improve working conditions. The committee had put together a long list of issues for Michael to raise at his first meeting. Michael impressed his colleagues with his eloquence and drive, and he was popular. In a staff newsletter, *Flotsam,* one of the other registrars painted a picture of him at the time. 'Dark and handsome, suave and erudite, sophisticated and yet having the common touch. These are the characteristics of the ideal anaesthetist, and surprisingly here is a man with them all.'

Michael's father, Hedley, had taught him the 'Five Ps'—'prior preparation prevents piss-poor performance,' so he had learned to prepare for meetings carefully. Michael also picked up a few tips on negotiating from his dad and his articulate uncle, Justice Norman Jenkyn, a QC and later president of the appellate tribunal of the Church of England in Australia. Still, he felt apprehensive, because it was the first time he had lobbied anyone since his days at medical school when he was a student rep. He found the right room, opened the squeaky door, then sat down at a large round table. The fluorescent lights flickered, and two middle-aged men sat chatting. Michael introduced himself. 'As you know, I'm the staff rep. Last month the House Committee ran a staff survey, and it uncovered several issues. Many of these concerns have been going on for years. One is the poor quality of the hospital's food, which the former committee chair told you about, and another is the lack of staff toilets.'

Michael and the managers talked about ways of fixing the problems. After two hours of negotiating, they agreed on a plan to improve the hospital's food and build more staff bathrooms. Michael glanced at his watch and realised he was due in the operating theatre. He excused himself and sprinted to the lifts. While he waited for the lift, he reflected on the meeting. Pleased with the outcome, he realised he had enjoyed the cut and thrust of bargaining with the senior managers. He revelled in bringing about change and hoped he would one day use his advocacy skills to improve the treatment of pain.

Towards the end of 1968, Michael returned home to find a letter from Sydney University waiting for him in the letterbox. He ripped it open while unlocking the front door. As he read the letter, Michele arrived home. 'We're going to Montreal,' he beamed. 'Sydney Uni has awarded me a fellowship for a year. I can do my pain research with Philip Bromage!'

Michael's epic journey had begun, but bureaucratic roadblocks forced him to endure an anxious seven-month wait for a visa to work in Canada.

2

MONTREAL

MEDICINE at McGill was in its heyday in the late 1960s, and on Michael's first day at the university in July 1969, he felt 'like a kid in a lolly shop'. When he arrived in the downstairs foyer of the medical school, a four-storey sandstone building on top of a hill with picturesque views over the Saint Lawrence River, one of his new colleagues, the anaesthetist Dr Mike Burfoot, warmly welcomed him. A week earlier, old family friends who lived in Montreal, Don and Barb Westaway, greeted Michael and Michele at the airport and took them to their home. The Westaways suggested that Nuns' Island would be an ideal place to live. In the middle of the Saint Lawrence River, it was a stone's throw from McGill and several McGill colleagues lived there including Mike Burfoot and his wife, Ruth. Much to their delight, Michael and Michele quickly found an apartment on the island and moved in.

'I'll introduce you to Professor Bromage first because I know how eager you are to meet him,' Burfoot said. 'After all, it's the reason you've travelled here from the other side of the world.'

Philip Bromage was close to finishing a world-first study—testing how well an epidural anaesthetic reduced a patient's pain after an operation and improved other essential activities like coughing. He also pioneered the use of epidural pain relief for pregnant women during labour. Although Michael had given several epidurals at Royal North Shore Hospital, he had never treated women in the labour ward, so he was looking forward to learning the new technique from Bromage. So were anaesthetists from around the world, who flocked to McGill to learn from this pioneering researcher.

Burfoot stopped in front of an open door and knocked. A handsome man in his fifties looked up from his desk and smiled. 'Ah, this must be our visitor from Australia,' Professor Philip Bromage said in a polished English accent. Tall and slim, with neatly combed grey hair and wearing a dark grey suit, he strode across the office and shook Michael's hand.

'Welcome to McGill,' he said, then pulled out two chairs from the desk inviting Michael and Burfoot to sit down. The three men chatted about Bromage's ideas on quickly relieving a patient's pain after surgery to help them get back to normal as soon as possible. Bromage suggested that once he settled in, Michael should pair up with the surgeon, Dr Charlie Wright, to conduct some studies.

'Dr Wright is scheduled to operate on several patients who have diseased blood vessels in their legs. You could test the effects of postoperative epidural anaesthesia on blood flow and pain.'

Michael's skin prickled as they talked about the study. After an hour, Bromage looked at his watch and said he was due at another meeting.

After leaving Bromage's office, Burfoot took Michael on a tour of McGill's anaesthesia department. As he walked through the vast corridors, Michael glimpsed enormous laboratories. The high-tech equipment and teams of scientists doing experiments thrilled him. It was much more sophisticated than what he was accustomed to in Australia. Along the way, he met several professors who chatted with him about their studies. Some of them were world leaders in pain research—he had read their journal articles. Burfoot introduced Michael to Charlie Wright, and they arranged to meet the following day to start planning their study.

At lunchtime, Michael bumped into Gordon Robson, the professor who had helped to organise his trip to McGill. Robson invited him to his laboratory later in the afternoon.

During the tour, Burfoot showed Michael the tunnels connecting different buildings at McGill. Michael had noticed a similar underground tunnel network in downtown Montreal that connected the metro system with various parts of the city. He thought this underground city, bursting at the seams with restaurants, cafes and shops, would be essential in the subzero temperatures of winter. He felt relieved that McGill University had its own underground tunnel network because it meant he wouldn't have to waste time putting on and taking off a heavy coat, hat and gloves every time he walked from one building to another during winter.

Three weeks after arriving at McGill, Michael and Wright started their study. As Michael walked into the icy-cold operating theatre, he felt elated but nervous. He shuddered as he realised the enormity of what he was doing—starting his first scientific study in the world's top centre for research on epidural anaesthesia.

After chatting with his patient, Michael sedated her. She was in her sixties and had varicose veins in her right leg. Once the patient was asleep, Wright made a slit in her right calf. He removed the diseased blood vessels, replacing them with healthy tissue to form a graft. Fifteen minutes later, Michael measured the amount of blood flowing through the graft and shin muscles. He also hung a thermometer on the patient's right big toe to check the skin temperature of her foot.

After another fifteen minutes, Michael injected local anaesthetic into the patient's epidural space, then repeated the same measurements. He found the amount of blood flowing through the graft had dramatically increased.[6] This result delighted Michael and Wright and they were curious about what had caused it. They repeated the procedure on seven more of Wright's patients, discovering similar reactions.

In late 1969, at the same time as Michael's study was reaching its peak, Michele and Michael's first son, James, was born. Michele had prepared by doing Lamaze classes that taught breathing, yoga, massage and other techniques to ease labour pain. Still, Michael anxiously hovered around her bedside while she was in labour and was relieved that Philip Bromage gave

Michele an epidural anaesthetic to ease her pain. So was Michele, although in those days the dose of local anaesthetic was extremely high, and Michele wasn't keen on the side effects—loss of sensation and movement in her legs. But she felt honoured that the father of epidural anaesthesia was her anaesthetist. 'Phillip kept doing pin-prick tests to see what I could feel up and down my leg. Which I didn't mind because it gave him good data for his research.'[5]

Once Michael and Michele took James home, he turned their lives upside down because he had colic and woke constantly. Michael got up through the night to change James' nappy, but his tiny baby slept fitfully, and he ended up pacing around the apartment as he tried to settle his son. It was the middle of winter and snowing almost daily. Michele found it challenging to cope with the intensity of Montreal's arctic conditions and being confined inside the apartment all day with a newborn. It was a tough time for her as she adjusted to life as a new mother in a foreign country without family and old friends around her. Overseas phone calls were expensive, and letters took weeks to arrive from Australia, so she couldn't rely on them to ease her homesickness. Still, her parents had taught her to make the best of difficult situations, so she soldiered on. She would later instil the same values in her children.

Following James' birth, Michael and Charlie Wright wrote a journal article describing how blood flow through a vascular surgical graft increased with improved pain relief—a revolutionary concept at the time—and they submitted it to the journal, *Surgery, Gynecology and Obstetrics*.[6] It was the first time Michael had written an article for a medical journal, so he was excited but impatient to hear a response from the journal. Wright had explained that long delays lasting more than a year were a normal part of the publishing process, so Michael knew they would have to wait several agonising months before the journal would contact them.

Michael was on call two nights each week, but he tried to arrive home early every other night so he could help Michele with James. During winter he caught two buses to McGill because so much salt was used on Montreal's snowy roads that the city was notorious for rusted cars.

One night on the way home, the first bus dropped him off at a bus stop. It didn't have a shelter, so he had to wait in the frigid air for the second bus. But the bus was delayed. He waited and waited, and the chill enveloped him, penetrating deep into his bones. Drawing his heavy wool coat tightly around him, he stamped his numb feet to keep warm. The tip of his nose felt like an icicle, and his vaporised breath formed a fog. 'It was way below zero. I had trouble breathing and was losing the feeling in my hands and feet despite jiggling them.' After what seemed an eternity, the bus turned up, and Michael returned home. As he walked through the front door and into the living room, he absorbed the warmth, and feeling returned to his extremities. 'When Michele saw me, she thought something terrible had happened because a frightened-looking husband greeted her. She said I looked like a ghost.'

In Michael's application for the travelling fellowship to study in Montreal, he had proposed inserting electrodes into the epidural space of patients to provide pain relief. This technique was an early form of neuromodulation—alteration or modulation of nerve activity by delivering electrical stimulation or drugs directly to the nerve. To his great disappointment, the electrodes he needed for the procedure were not yet available. In 1967 an innovative neurosurgeon, Dr C. Norman Shealy, had inserted a single electrode at the end of a needle through a patient's epidural space into a cavity within the spine, but some fluid protecting the brain and spinal cord leaked out. Such a leakage can be dangerous, potentially causing a severe headache or even an infection such as meningitis or a brain abscess. Shealy wrote a paper about his study, but neurosurgery journals refused to publish it because it was so controversial. In the end, the journal *Anesthesia and Analgesia* published it.[7] Michael was keen to explore this unique technique, but he had a frustrating eight-year wait until the biotechnology company, Medtronic, first manufactured suitable electrodes.

Some weekends the Cousins stayed with the Burfoots at their hobby farm in Burlington, Vermont. Philip Bromage and his wife, Meg, also had a farm in Northern Vermont and Michael and Michele stayed with them too. Before the Cousins had arrived in Montreal, Meg Bromage was involved in a car accident during a visit to England. Tragically as she sat on the side of the road after the accident she was hit by a passing car, severely injuring her leg. She languished in an English hospital for some time, so Bromage took her back to Canada. When they arrived home, Bromage took her to the Royal Vic, McGill University's hospital, hoping the highly skilled medical team could help her.

The hospital's most experienced orthopaedic surgeon examined her leg, then shook his head. He told her it was so grievously injured he had no other option but to amputate it. Afterwards, Meg struggled with intense phantom limb pain. Sadly, although she had access to the best pain specialists in Montreal, including Professor Ronald Melzack, a famous McGill psychologist who had a particular interest in phantom pain, no-one could relieve her unrelenting pain. Michael worried about Meg and searched his journals for clues on how to reduce phantom limb pain. So did Bromage, but at the time little was known about it.

During his year in Montreal, Michael worked full-time as an anaesthetist at the university hospital and did double shifts so he could use his day off to research acute postoperative pain. Acute pain is the body's warning system that tissue damage has occurred, and it usually settles once the injured tissues have healed. Most doctors at McGill believed that chronic pain—pain that lasts longer than three months—was just a prolonged form of acute pain. But one day at McGill when Michael chatted with the British neuroscientist, Professor Patrick Wall, the eminent researcher explained that different mechanisms in the nervous system cause acute and chronic pain. Wall, who was tall and skinny, said if acute pain was poorly managed, it could transition to chronic pain. 'And chronic pain is so complex it is diabolically difficult to treat,' he added. Michael also regularly bumped into Ronald Melzack, the famous McGill psychologist, and they discussed the differences between acute and chronic pain. In one of their exchanges, Melzack told him that feeling anxious or tired could increase a person's chronic pain, a new idea at the time.

As Michael mulled over his conversations with Melzack and Wall, he realised many of his patients at Royal North Shore Hospital had suffered from chronic pain. He felt a pang of guilt that he hadn't been able to reduce their suffering. A raft of questions raced through his mind. *Why does acute pain sometimes transition to chronic pain? What treatments work? If they work, why?* He resolved to find the answers while in Montreal.

Melzack and Wall had proposed the revolutionary Gate Control Theory of Pain in 1965, four years before Michael visited McGill.[8] The two researchers had sketched their original idea on a cocktail napkin in a Boston bar several years earlier. In 1962, they wrote an article describing their concept and published it in the prestigious journal *Brain*.[9] But Wall often told his colleagues that only three people ever read it.

Over the following months, they wrote another paper, developing their ideas with each new draft. The journal *Science* published 'Pain Mechanisms: a new theory,' in 1965.[8] Melzack later said some researchers loved it but most hated it.[10]

Melzack and Wall believed something occurred in the spinal cord and at other levels of the nervous system to alter the processing of pain signals. Contrary to other pain researchers, they thought pain signals flowed in two directions through the nervous system—from the injured area of the body up the spinal cord to the brain, then back down the spinal cord to the damaged tissues. This idea contradicted one of the original theories of pain proposed by the French philosopher and mathematician, René Descartes, in the seventeenth century.[11] Descartes claimed pain signals flowed in one direction from the body to a dedicated pain centre in the brain and the intensity of pain was directly related to the amount of associated tissue injury.[12] This theory left several questions unanswered, such as, what causes chronic pain and phantom limb pain?

Melzack and Wall suggested that 'nerve gates' in the spinal cord controlled the flow of pain signals to the brain. Excitatory chemicals in the nervous system opened the gates, increasing the intensity of the pain, and inhibitory chemicals closed the gates, turning down the volume of pain. Melzack and Wall thought that if a person felt stressed or anxious, the nervous system released excitatory chemicals, opening the gates and intensifying the pain. But if a person was calm and relaxed, the nervous system released inhibitory chemicals, closing the gates and reducing the pain.

BREAKING THROUGH THE PAIN BARRIER

If correct, the Gate Control Theory opened several alternative treatment approaches for chronic pain because it considered psychological factors such as depression and anxiety that can alter the way the nervous system processes pain signals. Most doctors dismissed the mental health issues linked with chronic pain, classifying them as 'reactions to pain'. They routinely labelled patients with persistent back pain as 'crocks' before sending them to a psychiatrist.

One afternoon at McGill, Patrick Wall gave a lecture on the Gate Control Theory to a group of neuroscientists and doctors. The seminar room was stiflingly hot, and the grey upholstered chairs crammed close together because so many people had packed into the high-ceilinged space. Michael sat spellbound as Wall, who was bald on top of his head and wore a beard and largish glasses, meticulously described existing concepts of pain, then tore them apart. The room erupted as Wall's colleagues reacted to his provocative claims that pain signals flowed in two directions and could be altered in the spinal cord and brain.

As Michael listened to the lecture, he realised pain would one day be a mainstream field of medicine. Pain medicine as a profession was in its infancy, and it lacked the resources needed to make breakthrough discoveries about new treatments for pain. It wasn't a 'sexy' area, but pain medicine intrigued Michael. Patrick Wall opened his eyes to the fast-approaching explosion in knowledge about pain and its treatment, and Michael's mind raced with possibilities. He started thinking about research questions he hadn't thought of before. As each question formed, he designed a study in his head. He knew it would stop him sleeping that night, but he didn't care because his ideas energised him. Still, he knew he needed to settle on one idea to research at a time if he was going to make any progress in breaking through the pain barrier.

On the nights that James settled, Michael and Michele sat on the sofa listening to records—classical music such Bach, Beethoven and Grieg. Michael also enjoyed jazz musicians such as Earl Hines, Louis Armstrong and Jelly Roll Morton. While listening to music, Michele read novels, and Michael studied articles about the latest developments in pain research. During the summer following James' birth, Poppy and Trenham visited, a wonderful boost to Michele's spirits. Geoff Cousins and his wife Gayle also came to stay after a business trip to New York.

Michael and Michele felt 'at home' living in Canada, possibly because it is a Commonwealth country like Australia. They struck up several close friendships and often shared lunches and dinners with friends on weekends. Michele appreciated the way Michael's colleagues and their wives took her and Michael under their wing while they lived so far from Australia with a tiny baby. In future years she would often invite Michael's overseas colleagues to her home for a meal when they visited Australia because she knew how hard it was to be alone in a new country.

One day Melzack and Wall were standing in an empty corner of the recovery room of the university hospital with Philip Bromage. They seemed more fired up than usual and were experimenting with a primitive-looking machine, a device the size of a doughnut that vibrated—an early version of the transcutaneous electrical nerve stimulation devices that Wall later co-invented and are so commonly used to relieve pain today.[ii] 'What's going on here today?' Michael asked. Melzack told him they thought the device might activate nerve fibres in the spinal cord that curbed the flow of pain signals.

'That day was the beginning of Melzack and Wall's attempts to test their Gate Control Theory,' Michael said. 'And it all unfolded from there. They were trying to see if their theory worked. Once they had confirmed its practical value, they wanted to create new treatments to improve chronic pain management. So did I.'

Melzack and Wall's original ideas inspired Michael. The pair described themselves as iconoclasts. Intensely excited by research, they 'lived and breathed it'. Michael enjoyed meeting people with a similar passion for medical science, and found it electrifying to spend time with his two colleagues. Patrick Wall could be intimidating at times, but Michael admired him—'he had a fierce intelligence, and his mind was razor sharp'. An avid birdwatcher in his spare time and a chain-smoker, Wall stridently articulated his left-wing views. His political leanings 'ruffled a few feathers' among the medical profession, but he ignored the criticism, brushing it aside. He was generous and provided financial support to several struggling artists and left-wing organisations. As well as co-inventing transcutaneous electrical nerve stimulation, Wall designed underwear elastic that gripped clothes, and hearing aids embedded in spectacle arms.

In contrast, Ronald Melzack, a Canadian, was gentle with everyone and 'had a special touch' according to Michael. 'He was extremely sensitive and very aware of everyone around him.' His warm smile and sparkling eyes endeared him to his colleagues and students—his students voted him as McGill's best instructor for several consecutive years and the awards lined his office walls. He was proud of them. When colleagues asked Melzack to provide feedback on his students, he made positive comments about them all, making it difficult to differentiate among them. In 1967, Melzack published a book for children, *The Day Tuk Became a Hunter and other Eskimo Stories*, including the legend of Sedna, an Inuit sea goddess.[13]

Early one Monday morning in February 1970, a McGill secretary phoned Michael. Her boss was the head of McGill's Department of Surgery, Professor Lloyd McLean. She invited Michael to a meeting with the professor that afternoon at the Royal Vic. He couldn't fathom why McLean, who was also Royal Vic's Surgeon-in-Chief, had requested a meeting.

On the dot of one o'clock after a snatched lunch, Michael headed to McLean's office. On the way, he mulled over the likely topics McLean would raise. He knocked on the dark wooden door and heard McLean call out for him to enter. Stepping in, Michael walked across the room and sat on one of the black leather chairs in front of the mahogany desk. Bookcases brimming with tomes lined the walls, and the intoxicating fragrance of lilies hung in the air. McLean thanked Michael for coming at such short notice. With a steady gaze, he asked Michael to anaesthetise one of his patients who was having a liver transplant the following day. Michael nodded and asked McLean about the patient.

'It's a gorilla.'

Michael gasped. 'A what?'

'I'm doing a liver transplant on a gorilla tomorrow morning,' McLean said calmly. 'I want you to anaesthetise it for me.'

'You can't anaesthetise a gorilla *here*,' Michael spluttered. The previous week he had heard rumours about one of the surgeons operating on a gorilla at the Royal Vic, but he brushed it off as a joke.

A silence settled between them.

McLean cleared his throat, then told Michael the gorilla, whom he had named Mr Gorilla because the animal required a temporary passport to travel from its home in a Los Angeles university laboratory, was downstairs in the basement. McLean explained his plans for the following day and asked Michael to get everything ready.

'See you at eight o'clock sharp,' McLean said abruptly, standing up to signal the end of the meeting.

Michael left the office, striding down the corridor to consult his colleague, the eminent anaesthetist, Dr Earl Wynands. Michael admired Wynands, whose 'true gentlemanly manners' reminded him of his father, Hedley. Wynands struggled to see because macular degeneration had destroyed his vision. But he had never seriously considered quitting medicine.

'I knew I was very good at my job and I had help whenever I needed it,' Wynands said in an interview. 'I always had a technician or a resident with me during operations, so I knew the patients were not at risk because of my eyesight.'[14] To compensate for his fading vision, Wynands bent close to his patients while administering anaesthesia and relied on his highly developed sense of touch.

Michael stepped into Wynands' office, closed the door, checking it was locked. Still standing and in a hushed voice, he explained his predicament. He asked Wynands to assist him during the surgery. Wynands nodded, a wry smile spreading across his face. He suggested Michael take a seat because they had a long afternoon ahead of them planning the procedure.

'Tomorrow might determine whether or not I go on in research or onto anything at all,' Michael muttered as he sat down.

The following morning, Michael's eyes flew open. He had a knot in the pit of his stomach. At first, he couldn't work out what was troubling him, but then he remembered McLean had booked Mr Gorilla for surgery at nine o'clock. And Michael was the anaesthetist! He felt mightily relieved that Earl Wynands had agreed to assist him, but it couldn't quell his feeling of trepidation.

Michael caught two buses to the Royal Vic. The closer he got to the hospital, the more his sense of foreboding intensified. He met up with Wynands and McLean in the foyer and McLean introduced him to a short man, who turned out to be an animal handler. The trio followed McLean down steep concrete stairs to the lower basement. No-one spoke. The only sound was the squelching of the animal handler's rubber shoes. But once they reached the basement, Michael could hear a thunderous banging noise and shrieking. A bubble of fear rose in his chest. He noticed McLean quicken his pace as they approached the racket. It reached a crescendo as McLean opened a heavy dark door. Michael peeked inside before stepping into the room. He flinched as he glimpsed the raging gorilla crashing against the sides of the cage.

'I got the fright of my life,' Michael admits. 'The deafening bang, bang, bang was menacing.'

At first, he remained close to the door, ready for a quick escape, but as the animal handler calmed Mr Gorilla, Michael edged closer to the cage. The four men chatted about the procedure, then Michael pulled on gloves and a green surgical gown. His throat tightened as he lifted the needles and anaesthesia from his black leather bag. Taking a deep breath, he filled a tranquilliser gun with a 'Curare-like drug' that would paralyse the gorilla for fifteen minutes. It would also stop Mr Gorilla from breathing. Michael handed the device to the animal handler, who pointed it at the bulging muscle at the top of Mr Gorilla's right arm. He pulled the trigger. Within seconds, Mr Gorilla collapsed, groaning as he fell to the floor of his cage.

'From the moment we got the Curare in,' Michael said, 'we jumped into the cage, inserted a laryngoscope and breathing tube, then Earl started pumping air into the gorilla's lungs.'

Michael stepped backwards out of the cage. He glanced at McLean. 'So, what happens now?'

McLean grinned. 'We're taking him up to the operating theatres in the lift.'

'We're going up in the public lift?' Michael stammered.

'Yeah, I've organised it with the supervising sister,' McLean said nonchalantly. He poked his head out the door. 'The coast's clear,' he whispered. 'Let's get started.'

The four men lifted Mr Gorilla onto a trolley, covering him in a green surgical drape. They wheeled the trolley along the corridor to the lift with Wynands trotting alongside pumping air into the animal's lungs. The lift seemed to take an eternity to arrive. When it did, McLean and the animal handler pushed the trolley inside. The lift operator glanced at the green drape, glared at McLean, then shook his head. 'I'm not even going to ask you. I don't want to know.'

McLean, Wynands, the animal handler and Michael collectively held their breath as they watched the control panel light up at each floor. Michael kept his eyes fixed on the green drape to see whether Mr Gorilla showed any signs of regaining movement. A pungent, musky odour filled the tiny, enclosed space.

Suddenly, the lift stopped, and the doors jerked open. Before anyone could stop them, three people crammed into the lift—McLean had forgotten to bar the public from the lift while they transported their cargo. The three strangers peered at the draped trolley with a bemused look on their faces. Lloyd stared at the ceiling. Michael held his breath.

When they arrived at the right floor, they left the lift, relieved that no-one had questioned them about their patient. They headed for the operating theatres where a supervising nurse waited outside their allotted theatre. When she spotted them, she rolled her eyes and sighed, then directed the four men into the plaster room, where they planned to shave Mr Gorilla's thick fur.

'We had to do a lot of clipping,' Michael said. 'And fast! I was worried the effects of the drug would wear off before we were ready.'

Mr Gorilla looked skinny without his fur, but his muscles were massive. The trio prepared him for surgery with the help of the animal handler. But the animal stirred, sending a shiver of panic up Michael's spine.

Michael and McLean put a plaster cast on Mr Gorilla's arms and legs to immobilise them. 'It was the moment of truth, because if we hadn't given him enough sedation, he would've ripped us to pieces. I've never been as terrified in my life.'

Michael didn't want to hurt Mr Gorilla while he inserted the cannula for the general anaesthetic, so first, he injected local anaesthetic into the animal's right hand. He waited for the local anaesthetic to take effect, deftly inserted a cannula into Mr Gorilla's hand then started running doses of general anaesthetic through it.

'Mercifully, Mr Gorilla fell unconscious in an instant,' Michael said. 'I don't think I've ever felt more relieved in my life.'

Nine months after arriving in Montreal, Michael received a message from Philip Bromage—Louis Raines, the Editor-in-Chief of medical books at the publishing house J. B. Lippincott & Co. wanted to see him. Raines had heard about the young Australian pain researcher and travelled from Brooklyn to meet Michael. When Raines arrived at McGill and introduced himself, Michael was surprised by his strong Brooklyn accent—it was the first time he had heard it outside of Hollywood movies.

Raines asked Michael whether he would produce a textbook on local and regional anaesthesia, with an emphasis on pain. He explained that Michael would need to travel the world, talking to pioneering pain researchers about their findings. Michael was flattered and eagerly accepted the offer despite its daunting nature. He and Raines discussed possible co-editors. They needed someone from North America who was better known because Michael as a young Australian pain researcher didn't yet have a high profile. Having a prominent Northern American co-editor would help to attract talented contributors to cover all the areas of regional anaesthesia and pain that had to be included in the textbook. As Raines walked from the office he firmly shook Michael's hand, giving him his 'best poissonal regards'.

Michael and Michele had planned to return to Australia straight after their year in Montreal. But a few months before they were due to leave, Michael received a phone call from Professor John Bunker, Chair of Stanford University's Anaesthesia Department. Bunker had heard about Michael's research and offered him a role at Stanford as an assistant professor. Michele was excited but disappointed about changing the original plan to return to Australia after the twelve-month stint in Montreal. She was keen to go back to Sydney to spend time with her family and friends, but she agreed to move to Stanford for one year because she knew it was a tremendous opportunity for Michael to progress his pain research.

In July 1970, Michael, Michele and James left Montreal for the month-long drive to Stanford. Their car didn't have air-conditioning, and they travelled the five thousand kilometres from Montreal to California through blazing heat with 'a baby bouncing around in the back of the car'.[15] James started crawling one night in their motel room and from then on, instead of happily sitting in his car bed, a frustrated James tried to crawl across the back seat. Michele sat in the back of the car, trying to distract him from his mission, but he persisted, determined to practise his new skill.[5]

A few days before the Cousins family started their journey, Michael learned that the journal *Surgery, Obstetrics, Gynaecology* had prepared the proofs for his first paper on the effects of epidural anaesthesia on pain and blood flow after blood vessel surgery.[6] Charlie Wright had promised to send the proofs to a post office box in Calgary, so when the manuscript arrived in that city, Michael picked it up. He had goosebumps while he sat in the car reading it and regretted leaving his good friend, Charlie. The pair had struck up a tremendously strong research partnership, but Michael believed his next destination—Stanford University—'was an absolute powerhouse, as it still is'.

3

STANFORD

THE Cousins family arrived at Stanford University in late August 1970. Dionne Warwick's hit *Do you know the way to San José?* was on the car radio, and despite the five thousand kilometre drive, Michael and Michele felt exhilarated. Michael was impatient to start his new job, and before finding their home, they drove around the campus, marvelling at its beauty.

To Michele and Michele's surprise, tall eucalypts and palm trees lined the driveway, making them feel at home. After four weeks of driving from Montreal in the sweltering heat, they immediately relaxed. They decided to go past the modern house they would rent on the edge of Mountain View, nine kilometres from Stanford. They couldn't move in for another five weeks. But to their great relief, Michael's friend, the obstetric anaesthetist, Gordon Taylor, had invited Michael and Michele to stay with his family until the rental house was available.

Michael rode his bicycle to Stanford each day, relishing the opportunity to keep fit and ponder his research ideas. Once he had settled into his new job as an anaesthetist at the Stanford University Hospital, he planned to continue his studies on the effects of epidural anaesthesia on pain and blood flow. While in Montreal, Michael had often chatted with a

McGill surgeon, Professor Gutelius, about the toxicity of drugs commonly used as general anaesthetics. He had also attended several lectures in the surgery department. One of them was about kidney physiology and how anaesthetic drugs affected it. He was keen to know more and read journal articles on the topic. Gutelius told him that a Stanford anaesthetist, Richard Mazze, was studying the toxicity of methoxyflurane. He said Mazze was curious and driven and 'followed his nose' while researching. Gutelius suggested Michael meet the young Stanford professor.

Once Michael's roster at the hospital stabilised, he took a day off and met with Mazze. Mazze's parents were Jewish and migrated from Poland decades earlier. He had a boyish face and cheeky smile and had inherited his parent's dark hair and eyes. The first thing Michael noticed was Mazze's intense intellectual energy. Their conversation about methoxyflurane toxicity energised Michael, but it made him impatient to get started on his own investigation.

A few weeks later, he was in his office fossicking around in his bottom desk drawer. He had a bulging folder of the latest data on epidurals and blood flow that grew fatter every day, and was close to finishing the planning of his next study—an extension of the epidural anaesthesia research he and Charlie Wright had done at McGill. While Michael dug around looking for a particular journal article, Richard Mazze walked across to him.

'Would you like to join me on my methoxyflurane studies?' Mazze asked.

Michael was interested but determined to continue his studies on the effects of epidural anaesthesia on pain and blood flow. During the next few weeks, however, Mazze urged him to consider his offer. Michael was conflicted, unsure which direction to take. Mazze was so persistent that Michael delayed the start of his epidural research and instead ran some studies with Mazze on methoxyflurane toxicity.

Over the next couple of weeks, the two researchers planned their project. They wanted to know whether methoxyflurane was toxic to the kidney, and if so, why? Once they were ready, they spent long hours in the laboratory studying the effects of methoxyflurane on rats. This was a strange experience for Michael. He hadn't previously worked with small laboratory animals, but he appreciated the opportunity to learn a new skill. To give himself time to work in the lab, Michael spent a full day at the university hospital and then did a night shift. He took the next day off to do his research. This regimen was taxing, particularly when he started studying the effects of methoxyflurane on patients. It meant arriving at the hospital at five o'clock—even though Michael wasn't a 'morning person'— to get everything ready for the day.

The Stanford years were a busy time for Michael and Michele. They enjoyed living in California and spent weekends exploring national parks or sharing lunches and dinners with their friends from the hospital and university. Michael found a part-time job for Michele as a medical editor and Michele arranged for a registered daycare to mind James two afternoons each week while she edited research papers. In early 1972 Michele was due to deliver her second baby. She had again done Lamaze classes in preparation and felt confident to deliver her baby without an epidural. Their second son, Richard, arrived without fuss. Much to his parents' relief, once home, he quickly fell into a routine. Richard was an 'angelic' baby, breastfeeding well, sleeping soundly and always happy. Of course at the time, no-one could have imagined what the future would hold for him.

When Richard was a few months old, Michael flew to Seattle to meet John J. Bonica, the formidable 'Grand Man' of pain medicine. Michael had longed to meet Bonica ever since studying the professor's pain textbook in Sydney University's medical school library. He was keen to seek the professor's advice on the outcomes of his epidural anaesthesia and blood flow study.

Bonica was driven to improve pain management. Following the Second World War, he had cared for injured soldiers returning from the front with severe pain. The war veterans' pain problems were so complex Bonica quickly realised his skills as an anaesthetist were inadequate to treat them. Instead, he thought the veterans needed help from a team of doctors from different fields. He empathised with the war veterans because he too suffered from unrelenting pain after a career as a professional wrestler while a medical student. His income from wrestling had funded his studies but left him with agonising back injuries. Over the years, he endured twenty-two back operations, but sadly, none reduced his suffering.

In 1947, Bonica set up a pain centre in Washington State, staffed by doctors from various medical specialties.[16] This approach was an early version of what would later become known as interdisciplinary pain management—a combination of specialist medical, psychological, physiotherapy and other professional services to address the multiplicity of issues faced by people living with pain.

Later, Bonica launched a pain clinic at the University of Washington in Seattle. Every Friday at noon, a team of specialist physicians would meet to discuss the patients with chronic pain they had seen during the week. The week Michael visited the University of Washington, he took part in a Friday meeting. Shortly before midday, doctors streamed into the conference room at the University of Washington pain centre and sat around a large rectangular table. The energy level was high as the doctors chatted; their pagers beeped incessantly. At precisely twelve o'clock, Bonica strode in. Michael sat at the end of the table in the visitor's chair. As Bonica lowered himself into his chair, a hush fell over the room. One by one, doctors spoke about the patients they had assessed that week. Michael perched on the edge of his seat, in awe of the speakers. He was astonished to hear anaesthetists, rehabilitation specialists, neurologists, psychiatrists and rheumatologists all discuss the same patients. It was the first time he had witnessed a team approach to managing chronic pain, sparking his interest in pursuing interdisciplinary pain management.

McGill and Stanford colleagues had warned Michael that Sicilian-born Bonica had a dominant personality and was a force to reckon with. Michael was apprehensive about his first one-on-one meeting with the professor, scheduled later on. 'I was afraid I'd say something stupid, or that John Bonica would think I was wasting his time.'

All too soon, four o'clock arrived. Michael knocked on Bonica's door, hesitating for a few seconds after Bonica called out to him to enter. He squared his shoulders, then opened the door. Oak bookshelves filled to overflowing with thick textbooks and rows of medical journals lined the office walls. Bonica rose to greet Michael. 'John wasn't very tall, but he had massive hands and a steel grip. I felt my bones would break if he had squeezed my hand any harder,' Michael recalls. Bonica wore his 'characteristic uniform'; a three-piece suit with gold watch chains suspended from the waistcoat and gold-rimmed glasses. Bonica's stocky build astonished Michael. 'His broad shoulders were almost as wide as his height, and his enormous chest looked as hard as a rock.'

During the meeting, Bonica 'listened with apparent irritation' to Michael's research findings, 'firing off a series of staccato questions'. Michael wondered whether this meant the professor didn't approve of the research study or its results. At the end of the meeting, Bonica's response indelibly imprinted itself in Michael's memory: 'Not bad, son. Keep up the excellent work.' As Michael stood up to leave, Bonica's parting words encouraged him. 'Always get your facts right, son. And never, never give up.'

Michael returned to Stanford looking forward to continuing his research. He and Mazze were close to completing their methoxyflurane study, and Michael was living on adrenaline. A few months after arriving home from Seattle, Mazze and Michael sat side-by-side in the brightly lit lab reviewing the results of their study. Benches covered in sophisticated measuring equipment surrounded them. Almost at the same moment, they looked across at each other.

'This data shows that methoxyflurane is toxic to the kidney at the doses anaesthetists use during surgery,' Mazze said, his voice an octave higher than usual.[17]

Michael nodded. 'It looks like the liver breaks it down into by-products that do the damage.'

Although methoxyflurane was a popular general anaesthetic, Michael knew many anaesthetists and surgeons didn't like it because it remained active in the body for so long after surgery. He was sure they would like it even less when they heard it caused potentially lethal kidney damage in some patients.

Mazze and Michael conducted several more studies and once they were certain their findings were correct, they set out to ensure the

American Government banned methoxyflurane from operating theatres.[18] First, they met with representatives from the Food and Drug Administration, thinking it would ban the drug. But the FDA managers refused to act. Then Michael and Mazze discussed their conclusions with the American Medical Association and pharmaceutical industry leaders. The executives at these meetings were openly hostile, criticising the results. Undeterred, Mazze and Michael continued their campaign, using every opportunity to lobby decision-makers. Several influential individuals and organisations fiercely contested their findings, but the two researchers battled on, despite the mounting pressure.

Michael had learned from his father Hedley the importance of showing leadership and resilience under challenging circumstances. When his confidence flagged during the methoxyflurane struggle, he drew reassurance from the way his father always fought for what he believed was right. His mother too was an energetic campaigner, acting as a vocal advocate in her role as president of Royal North Shore Hospital's volunteer association.

Michael enjoyed taking part in the methoxyflurane study. He believes the rigour that went into it was a significant learning experience for him. It also kindled his interest in pharmacology as a broad subject and toxicity because: 'no drug is useful unless it has a sufficient margin between safe and toxic doses'.

During the late 1960s and early 1970s, an informal movement of doctors, allied health professionals and scientists who were interested in pain medicine formed around John Bonica. Bonica yearned to encourage basic researchers—who conduct experiments in the laboratory—to team up with clinical researchers, whose research focuses on patients. He believed these collaborations would speed up the development of new treatments. Bonica waited until the pain medicine community had built up a head of steam, then in late May 1973, made his move. He invited pain professionals from around the world to a meeting in a former nunnery in Issaquah, a suburb thirty kilometres to the east of Seattle. To his surprise, over three hundred leading lights of the pain world from thirteen countries arrived to take part.[16] One hundred prominent pain researchers and clinicians presented papers. The delegates unanimously agreed to set up an international organisation devoted to pain research and treatment. They named it the International Association for the Study of Pain (IASP).[19]

Michael was on duty at Stanford University Hospital during the Issaquah conference and was bitterly disappointed to miss it. But several colleagues who took part told him the mood at the event was electrifying. Their rapture was contagious, and Michael vowed to get involved in the new organisation.

At an early stage of his term at Stanford, Michael's colleagues regarded him as a future leader. The neurosurgeon, Professor John Loeser, kept hearing about a young Australian doctor who was impressing his Stanford colleagues. He said they viewed Michael as a rising star. 'Whenever anaesthetists were snooping around thinking about potential committee chairs, Michael's name popped up. He was on everyone's shortlist because he was hard-working, easy to get along with, and going up in the world.'[20] Professor Kathleen Foley, a neurologist at New York's Sloan Kettering Institute, agrees. When she first met Michael, Foley noticed he was a 'take charge' type of person. She also thought he was handsome with his glossy dark hair and chiselled cheekbones. Foley admired Michael's leadership skills and determination to understand the science of pain—to help him figure out what caused it. She also respected the way he did everything in his power to relieve his patients' pain and give them the best possible care.[21]

Michael's workload rose as he took on extra commitments and his reputation grew within the pain medicine community. In his meeting with John Bonica, the professor had shared a tip with him for tackling a demanding schedule. Bonica dearly loved his wife Emma, three daughters and son, and was adroit at balancing family time with a punishing workload.

'You don't have to end the day after dinner,' Bonica said. 'Enjoy a little snooze after reading your kids a bedtime story and tucking them into bed. Then after the nap, write late into the night.' Michael followed this advice to give him time to start work on his pain textbook.

Towards the end of 1973, the head of Stanford's anaesthesia department invited Michael to extend his appointment at the university. Michael and Michele discussed the opportunity late into every night for over a week. Michael wanted to 'repay' his Montreal travel fellowship by returning to practice in Australia. But he felt tempted to remain at Stanford because he'd started treating patients who suffered from chronic pain. He was also running studies on acute pain after surgery. Michael and Michele revelled in California's lifestyle, and Michele liked her job as a medical editor. The balance was overwhelmingly in favour of staying at Stanford because opportunities for academic research in anaesthesia in Australia were 'virtually nil'.

However, the couple felt the powerful tug of home. Michael believes 'a little bell rings in the breasts of Australians when they are away from their motherland. Eventually, it becomes too strong to ignore'. In the end, they decided to return to Australia so they could spend time with their ageing parents. They also wanted their children to grow up in Australia, close to their grandparents and cousins.

After launching his research career in North America, Michael wanted to continue it in Australia. 'I thought it would be a terrible waste to go into private practice because I'd already done five years of research, and the ball was rolling.' He yearned for a role in Australia that would enable him to combine clinical practice and research. He wrote a letter to the superintendent of Royal North Shore Hospital enquiring about job opportunities. To his delight, the superintendent offered him a position as a consultant anaesthetist and head of the hospital's nascent pain clinic.

Before he departed for Sydney, Michael served as a visiting professor at the Mason Clinic in Seattle. While there, he worked with the anaesthetist and pain medicine specialist, Dr Philip Bridenbaugh. Bridenbaugh was five years older than Michael and had gained valuable experience when he worked at the University of Washington with John Bonica. A distinguished pain researcher, he specialised in regional anaesthesia. During the visit Michael asked Bridenbaugh to partner with him on producing his textbook. Bridenbaugh enthusiastically accepted the invitation and so began a productive multi-decade partnership. The pair created an outline for each chapter, then invited experts from Australia and around the world to write them. Simultaneously, they embarked on a frenetic schedule of weekend conferences to explore the latest developments in pain medicine and regional anaesthesia. In the early 1970s, pain research had captured the imagination of scientists. This explosion in knowledge exhilarated Michael, but he had to 'run extremely fast' to keep up with the latest insights.

At Stanford, Michael had seen firsthand the immense value added to patient care by integrating treatment and scientific research. Interacting with the giants of pain medicine had reinforced his drive to pursue excellence and learn from the very best—two of his lifelong traits. He'd found several distinguished role models to guide him, and he took every opportunity to learn from them. The standards Melzack, Wall and Bonica set naturally came to be the standards Michael embraced.

'It was a fortunate convergence of three extraordinary individuals,' he said. 'My years in North America were like nothing else I've experienced through the rest of my life.'

4

THE TUG OF HOME

IN December 1973, two months after Queen Elizabeth II opened the Sydney Opera House, the Cousins returned to Sydney. They had toured the skeleton of the Opera House shells before departing Australia and were thrilled to see it completed. The building's mesmerising white tiled sails intrigued them. At first, the family stayed with Michele's parents, Poppy and Trenham, at their holiday house. Within a month they found a place of their own in Pymble, on Sydney's leafy upper North Shore. It was also close to both sets of grandparents and Royal North Shore Hospital.

The hospital's anaesthesia department was on an ancient verandah in an older section of the hospital. Intensive care units didn't exist at the time, so Michael cared for critically ill patients in the ward. Michael was determined to continue the research he had started in North America. At McGill and Stanford, he had learned to identify a clinical problem, design a research study to explore the issue, then apply insights gained from the research to patient care. However, his conviction to operate this way made for constant battles with the hospital's bureaucracy.

Different departments managed research and the treatment of patients, and administrators refused to change this approach. Michael stood up to his bosses and didn't yield, eventually gaining the funding to begin some research projects on top of working as a full-time anaesthetist. This persistence was an early indication of his tendency to dig in and fight when roadblocks obstructed the pursuit of his vision.

Shortly after moving to Pymble, Michael invited Louis Raines from J. B. Lippincott & Co. to dinner. Raines was visiting Sydney on business from New York and was keen to hear how work was progressing on the pain textbook Michael was co-editing with Philip Bridenbaugh. After dinner, in the family room, Raines started scratching his arms and legs. The scratching intensified throughout the evening, and Michael noticed red blotches on his guest's arms. When he asked him if he was okay, Raines assured Michael he was fine.

A few days later, Raines told Michael the red patches were flea bites. Michael was mortified. Michele did some detective work and discovered the previous owners of the house had a flea-ridden dog. Every time the two men met in later years, Raines asked Michael to give his 'best poissonal regards' to Michele, and they had a chuckle about the flea episode.

Michele and Michael enjoyed bushwalking, so on weekends they often took James and Richard on easy walks through the Ku-ring-gai National Park, close to their home. They also took them to Palm Beach and walked up to Barrenjoey Lighthouse. While there they taught their young boys how to ride a boogie board. Michael also sprinted along the beach and bodysurfed, taking him back to his days as a schoolboy athlete. During the week he squeezed exercise into his busy schedule by walking up the stairs at the hospital rather than taking the lift. One thing that drove him was the delight he experienced when helping patients regain their pre-injury activity levels, often after years of immobility because of chronic pain.

In early 1974, John Bonica telephoned Michael, inviting him to become Vice-President of the International Association for the Study of Pain's Asia–Pacific Region. Michael was flattered but hesitated. 'I'm very busy,' he said. 'I've only just returned from America and started a new job. I'm also working on the textbook, so I shouldn't take on too much more.'

Bonica was indignant. 'Listen, son. Are you going to do it? Yes or no?'

'I think I'd better do it.'

Michael said that was how John Bonica recruited all the association's office-bearers. 'Not one person was game to turn him down.'

Later in 1974, Richard Mazze rang Michael. He said several countries had banned methoxyflurane from operating theatres. Michael was ecstatic. The scientific papers the two researchers had published detailing the relationship between methoxyflurane and kidney toxicity had rocked the anaesthesia world.[17] [18] Mazze and Michael's courage, doggedness and willingness to fight for something they believed in had borne fruit. Michael had found the experience intensely stressful but a valuable learning opportunity, one he would draw on in future years.

During his first year back in Sydney, Michael heard that Flinders University in Adelaide was advertising for a Foundation Professor of Anaesthesia and Intensive Care for its new hospital and medical school. This was the first chair of its kind in Australia. Flinders University, in Adelaide's southern suburbs, had opened in 1966. At first, the university lacked a medical school and teaching hospital. But the area's rapidly growing population urgently needed its own acute care hospital rather than relying on Royal Adelaide Hospital, sixteen kilometres away. The South Australian Government decided to build a medical school within a new hospital, naming it Flinders Medical Centre. In the 1970s, this was considered innovative and forward-looking. The partially completed hospital and medical school were due to open the following year.

Although the role piqued his interest, Michael didn't apply for it, believing that at thirty-five years of age, he was too inexperienced to be a full professor. Still, by this early stage of his career he had published thirty-six scientific papers[22] and had been awarded a Doctorate in Medicine for the research he conducted with Richard Mazze on the toxicity of inhaled anaesthetics.[23] When Michael told his former boss, Professor Tom Reeve, he didn't intend to pursue the role, the senior surgeon urged him to reconsider. Flinders Medical School's Dean, Professor Gus Fraenkel—an advocate for anaesthetists—also encouraged him to apply.

Convinced he wouldn't be successful, Michael posted his application. A few weeks later he flew to Adelaide for an interview. When he returned to Sydney, he felt sure he wouldn't get the job. But the following week, and to his immense surprise, Flinders University offered him the position. Although elated, the responsibility and effort required to build an anaesthesia service and pain centre from scratch daunted him. He resolved to create a pain centre like the one he had witnessed at the University of Washington. 'I realised it was going to be quite a test, but I was up for the challenge.'

The new medical school at Flinders was still under construction when Michael started his new job, so he could influence the design of the operating theatres, ensuring they met the needs of anaesthetists and surgeons. He also lobbied for research laboratories and an animal house for laboratory animals such as rats and guinea pigs. For the first six months, he combined his new role at Flinders Medical Centre with his existing one at Royal North Shore Hospital. Every few weeks he flew to Adelaide for meetings that started early in the morning and ended late at night. He was tremendously enthusiastic and felt he was taking a significant step forward in applying what he had learned in North America to the advancement of pain medicine in Australia.

During the period Michael was commuting to Adelaide, Michele gave birth to the couple's third son, Jonathan, at Royal North Shore Hospital. After the birth, Michael worried about Michele's health. She had left hospital suffering from chickenpox and mastitis. To top it off, she ended up with shingles. Fortunately, a friend agreed to buy the family's house, removing one worry. Michele didn't relish the idea of moving to Adelaide so soon after returning from America and felt heartbroken to be leaving her family and friends again. At the same time, she loved the critical role she played in supporting Michael's quest.

In those days, many Sydneysiders thought of South Australia's capital city as a large country town rather than a city. International air services were yet to arrive there, and Adelaide was famous for its old sandstone churches and elite private schools.[24] But change was afoot, and it would profoundly impact Michael.

In 1970, South Australians elected a progressive Labor Government intent on reforming social policy. In an election policy speech, Don

Dunstan, South Australia's then Opposition Leader, laid out his vision if elected. 'South Australia will become the technological, the design, the social reform and the artistic centre of Australia…We'll set a standard of social advancement that the whole of Australia will envy.'[25] Within a few years of being elected, Dunstan's government had radically reformed environmental, consumer protection, racial discrimination, women's and Indigenous policy.

The Cousins arrived in Adelaide on a sizzling day in late 1975. It was forty degrees Celsius and South Australia was in the grip of a week-long heatwave. The state's residents sweltered at night, with temperatures often remaining in the thirties. Michael had arranged for the family to move into the new nurses' quarters at Flinders University until they bought a house. The accommodation lacked air-conditioning, and they struggled with the heat. Poppy arrived soon after to help Michele, who still suffered from shingles and appreciated her mother's support. Michele searched for a house on a slope, not wanting to live in a flat area hemmed in on three sides by neighbours' fences. But she found it challenging to find a house she liked in a hilly area. After five months of squatting in the nurses' quarters, a parent from James' school rented the Cousins her beach house at Glenelg, Adelaide's favourite seaside destination. Michael was embarrassed that his family had remained in the nurses' quarters for so long and he 'felt mightily relieved to leave'.

After six months of fruitless house hunting, Michele discovered the gracious National Trust house, 'Highfield,' in the quiet eastern Adelaide suburb of St Georges, twenty minutes from Flinders Medical Centre in good traffic. Its walls were fifty-three centimetres thick, and when the family stepped through the front door, the temperature inside was ten degrees cooler than outside. Michael set up a study in the one carpeted room of the huge basement. Sunshine streamed in from casement windows, making him feel less cut off from the outside world while he was down there. And it was 'beautifully quiet, the perfect place to work on weekends'.

Highfield soon became a hub for Michael's international and local pain medicine colleagues. He and Michele often invited colleagues for a home-cooked dinner—usually roast lamb or chicken. Sometimes Michael asked them at the last minute without giving Michele much notice. But she was adept at quickly rustling up a superb meal, and always kept supplies in the pantry to whip up a chocolate mousse or crème caramel. She would pre-cook dishes and store them in the freezer for emergencies. 'So if Mike said, "Oh gee, we should have so and so for a meal," I could pull out first, second and third course in an instant. I loved doing it because I had always appreciated being invited to colleagues' homes when we lived overseas.'

Michele revelled in the opportunity to meet talented researchers from across the globe who, like Michael, were striving to break through the pain barrier. Michael sincerely appreciated Michele's contribution to his life's work and often thanked her. 'Michele was instrumental in helping me to consolidate my career by helping me build my professional network.'

5

NURTURING A FLEDGLING

THE camaraderie among the medical school's professors impressed Michael when he arrived at Flinders University in 1975. They all 'camped' close together in cubicles in the library because tradesmen were still fitting out the medical school—an ideal way, Michael thought, for the new professors to get to know each other and start collaborating on research. He knew he would need their support to fund the pain centre.

From the outset, one of Michael's top priorities was to build a pain clinic and conduct pain research to improve the management of acute, chronic and cancer pain. But he constantly battled for funding, and the initial conviviality evaporated when the time came to negotiate with hospital administrators for resources. 'We were all great friends slapping each other on the back when we abutted on each other in the library,' Michael recalls. 'But when it came the time for cut and dice, it was every man for himself. I'd seen nothing quite like it. I was new at the game and still learning the ropes; I knew I needed to ramp up my efforts a hundredfold.'

At a breakfast meeting soon after Michael arrived at Flinders, he announced his plans to set up an interdisciplinary pain centre. A senior surgeon hissed, 'Over my dead body!' Everyone else looked down at the table, focusing on eating greasy croissants and sipping lukewarm coffee that tasted metallic from stewing too long in the urn. During his job interview, Michael had made clear his intentions to the interview panel, and by appointing him, he had assumed the hospital and university supported his plan to establish a pain centre as well as an anaesthesia service. Surprised and bitterly disappointed to meet so much resistance, he resolved to find a way through the roadblock.

Late one Sunday afternoon, a month after moving to Adelaide, Michael met with the hospital's administrators and other department heads. Eight men sat around a large rectangular table discussing funding submissions. It was stiflingly hot. Towards the end of the long meeting, they reached Michael's proposal. He had requested financial support from the university and hospital to build an interdisciplinary pain centre. One of the department heads snarled, 'Cousins, if you think you're going to walk out of this meeting with funding to set up a pain centre, you've got another think coming'.

A senior hospital bureaucrat said, 'Your brief is to create an anaesthetic service in the operating theatre and intensive care unit. Pain research and a pain clinic are not part of that brief'.

Undeterred, Michael dug in. He told the senior manager that access to pain management services was a fundamental human right. 'What price can you put on a person's quality of life?' he asked his colleagues. Some of his colleagues rolled their eyes. By the looks on their faces, Michael assumed they were thinking, 'Here he goes again'. The hospital and university administrators' response to Michael's funding submission would pay for 'one measly lecturer' and the equivalent of two anaesthetists. He reconciled himself to fighting for his 'share of the pie'.

Despite the hospital and university's lack of enthusiasm about Michael's plans, he persisted. He continued to search for the resources he needed to establish a pain centre. At first, he didn't have anywhere to locate a pain clinic, so he 'borrowed' a small area of the outpatients' department. His vigorous lobbying for anaesthesia research laboratories had paid off— the administrators offered him a generous space for them—so he used some of this allocation for the pain clinic and pain research.

Afternoons at Flinders were often frenzied because Michael tried to complete everything on his to-do list before running out the door. Sometimes he took part in meetings at night, but he assiduously tried to avoid them because he was committed to spending evenings with Michele and his children. 'It was a constant juggle. Team members would line up at my door wanting a "quick word" before I left for the day. I didn't want to hold up their research but getting home to my family was uppermost in my mind.' Still, he was often late for dinner, but at bedtime, he invented magical tales for his sons about the adventures of a rubber horse who flew all over the place. Each of his children still remember being enthralled by these stories. After tucking James, Richard and Jonathan into bed and kissing them good night, Michael headed to his study for a few hours of research or writing. Michele joined him because she was copyediting his textbook on pain and regional anaesthesia.

In 1975 the psychologist, Dr Ross Harris, joined Flinders Medical Centre in its community medicine department. Harris and Michael became friendly and often talked about the psychological impacts of chronic pain. Michael knew he should offer psychological services within the pain clinic, but he didn't have enough funding to pay for a psychologist. Harris, who had witnessed the benefits of cognitive behavioural therapy in patients with chronic pain during his time studying in America, offered to help. He suggested he treat patients in the pain clinic two days each week on a pro bono basis. Michael was ecstatic, gratefully accepting the generous offer.[26]

Flinders Medical Centre officially opened in April 1976. It was a year after Labor Prime Minister, Gough Whitlam, broadened access to Australia's health system by introducing Medibank, a national publicly funded health insurance system. Pain as a field of medicine was still in its infancy—it was just two years since John Bonica had launched the International Association for the Study of Pain, and the same year that the association started its journal *Pain*.

Michael got along well with many of his medical colleagues and often talked with them about the need to offer a team approach for managing chronic pain, lamenting his inability to do this because of inadequate funding. Some of his anaesthesia and psychiatry colleagues responded by offering their services on a pro bono basis—usually one or two days each week. 'I realised I would need to use my personal relationships to win over support and cobble services together. It came down to twisting arms and making my colleagues feel they could contribute. It was just a matter of goodwill.' Michael appreciated the generosity of the colleagues who volunteered their time to help him deliver pain services. But the treatments the pain clinic provided through the altruism of a few sympathetic supporters was a far cry from the premier interdisciplinary pain centre Michael dreamed of building.

Once he had raised the funds to pay them, one of Michael's top priorities was recruiting candidates for the Flinders' team. He did this by activating his professional networks and handpicking candidates with an impressive track record in research. One of the key attributes he sought was a passion for teaching because he wanted the scientists and clinicians to educate doctors and allied health professionals about pain. The pool of potential candidates with this combination of skills was minute.

Still, Michael was a good networker and continually searched for talented staff who shared his values. At first, white middle-class men dominated the team's makeup, as was the case across the medical world and academia. But Michael was committed to including women in the group. 'I can honestly say that every time I had an opportunity to get a woman appointed, that's what happened. It became easier when more women started to graduate from medical schools.' Over time, the diversity of recruits increased with the appointment of several senior women and researchers from Italy, Greece, Africa, the Middle East and Asia.

Michael encouraged the scientists to submit articles to prestigious journals to help them progress in their careers. He maintained a strict policy that his name would only appear on a paper when he had played a substantial role in the research. In these articles, he placed his name last to ensure his colleagues gained recognition for the publication. This practice was unusual among academics, but Michael wanted to help his colleagues advance their careers. He felt privileged to have spent time in North America learning from the world's top pain pioneers and felt he had a responsibility to mentor Australia's pain researchers.

Late in 1976 Michael travelled to Lisbon to take part in his first council meeting of the International Association for the Study of Pain. John Bonica had appointed Michael as a council member when he accepted the role of Vice-President of IASP Asia–Pacific. The council was a forum for the world's leaders in the nascent field of pain medicine to meet and exchange ideas. 'I felt like a neophyte among a group of giants. It was a wonderful experience for me as a junior person in this field to meet at firsthand the people whose papers I'd read.' Michael was delighted to see Patrick Wall and Ronald Melzack, and he enjoyed several conversations with them. But John Bonica was in hospital, having one of many back operations for injuries he had sustained during his professional wrestling career.[15]

When he returned to Adelaide after the council meeting, Michael stepped up his fundraising for the pain clinic. Despite being an intensely private person, he was the public face of pain medicine at Flinders and invested substantial time in raising money to support the pain centre's growth. But as a novice fundraiser, he struggled with this role. In a late-night phone call with John Bonica one weekend, Michael admitted his frustration.

'Search for funding in every nook and cranny,' Bonica advised. 'Even view patients as potential donors.' During that telephone conversation, Bonica surprised Michael by inviting him to become chair of IASP's finance committee. Michael was keen for the association to fund innovative research and education programs, but the fledgling organisation ran on a shoestring. He knew it would be a gargantuan struggle, but he was ready to rise to the challenge.

One of Michael's earliest appointments to the Flinders team was the Australian pharmacologist, Dr Laurie Mather. Mather had worked as a scientist in John Bonica's group at the University of Washington. Michael appointed Mather as Foundation Lecturer in Anaesthesia. This 'raised a few eyebrows' because Mather was a scientist rather than an anaesthetist, but Michael strongly believed his skill set was perfect. He didn't yield to pressure because he was confident in his choice.

For several months, Mather and the scientists he recruited worked in an empty laboratory because Michael lacked enough funds to purchase basic equipment such as microscopes, computers and software programs for analysing the data they collected in their studies.[27] Mather's team carried out applied pharmacology research on the effects of a drug on the body, and the complementary effects of the body on a drug. To do this, they needed reliable practical tools, such as gas-liquid chromatography for measuring minute quantities of drugs in blood samples.

Fortunately, Michael had brought a gas chromatograph with him from Sydney to restart his anaesthetic toxicity research. Whenever he or one of the scientists in his team wasn't using it, Mather borrowed it. But the device was in high demand, and Mather urgently required one for his laboratory.[27]

Once Michael raised enough funds to buy a second gas chromatograph, Mather's team studied the effects of pethidine on the body, and the body on the pethidine. They explored how these effects influenced pain control after surgery—work he had previously started while working in John Bonica's department in Seattle. Month by month, as they secured funds to purchase additional laboratory equipment, the researchers were able to undertake more complex investigations, giving the Flinders team answers to several questions, including why postoperative pethidine injections often provided inadequate pain relief.[27]

Weekends at home were busy. James was a talented athlete on the track and he also played Australian Rules football and later hockey. Michael or Michele would ferry him to training and matches and stay to watch him. Late on Saturday mornings, Michael would mow Highfield's lawn. The house was built on a three-quarter block of land, so it took nearly two hours to mow. 'Not much fun in scorching summer heat,' he recalls. Afterwards, Michele would carry a platter of salad vegetables and a jug of banana smoothie out onto the lawn for the family to enjoy a picnic lunch. One hot summer day, Michele told Michael she had to spend four hours each week sweeping up all the leaves in their garden. He knew she didn't like the never-ending chore, so he bought a device to vacuum the leaves. From then on, he assumed responsibility for leaf control—despite the racket made by the vacuum machine—because it gave him uninterrupted thinking time. On occasions, Michael also rescued Michele's favourite plants. One day Michele was worried one of them was dying, so Michael hooked up an intravenous drip. It survived, much to Michele's delight.

Early one morning, three of Michael's IASP council colleagues telephoned him from North America. They told him that since IASP's inception three years earlier, John Bonica had allowed Louisa Jones, who edited the University of Washington's anaesthesia research publications, to run the association on a part-time basis. However, as it grew, and the workload increased, Jones took on the role of full-time executive officer—pro bono. Suddenly, Bonica found himself without Jones' support at the University of Washington, prompting him to propose the association reimburse him for providing Jones' help. But several council members disagreed with this proposal. They told Michael that as chair of the association's finance committee, it was his responsibility to break the news to Bonica that they wouldn't repay him. Michael winced, apprehensive about Bonica's reaction. 'For a novice at my stage to approach the "Grand Man" with the decision was terrifying.'

On his next trip to Seattle for an IASP council meeting, Michael met with Bonica to inform him of the council's decision. They met in Bonica's office at the University of Washington. As Michael sat down, a silence fell between the two men. 'I was quaking in my boots because I thought John would eat me alive.' Their eyes locked across the vast desk. Squaring his shoulders, Michael told the professor the council's decision. His delivery was rapid and confident, but he felt a tight knot inside his stomach. A shadow crossed Bonica's face, and his eyes hardened. He stood up, pushing his chair back noisily. 'With smoke coming out of his nose, he walked around the desk to me, then placed his hand on my shoulder. The pressure under his hand intensified and became uncomfortable. I thought it would be the end of our relationship.' Unflinching and with Bonica still pressing down on his shoulder, Michael suggested several options, knowing his colleagues depended on him to resolve the issue. Bonica sighed, returned to his seat, and much to Michael's surprise, the two men amicably discussed the alternatives. They soon reached a compromise. 'I'll never forget it. Somehow, I came out of it without John chopping off both my hands and feet.'

Some of Michael's council colleagues were waiting outside Bonica's office, eager to see if Bonica had 'turned him into mincemeat'. To their amazement, Michael left the meeting unharmed.

Meanwhile, back in Australia, the Flinders research featured on the front page of the Adelaide afternoon newspaper *The News* on 8 November 1978 with the bold headline 'SA Team Smashes Pain Barrier'[28]—to the amusement of some of Michael's colleagues. The world's pain leaders were also taking notice of research papers on epidural pain relief published by the Flinders' scientists.[29] Kathleen Foley, head of the first pain service in an American cancer centre—the Memorial Sloan Kettering Cancer Center in New York City—closely watched the Flinders' research. The Sloan Kettering scientists often liaised with the Flinders researchers, and they adapted their studies in response to advice from the Adelaide group. The Flinders' team impressed Foley. She believed the scientists were at the cutting-edge in trying to understand what caused pain so they could develop new treatments.[21]

In August 1978, the International Association for the Study of Pain held its second world congress on pain in Montreal. Michael didn't attend because of commitments at Flinders Medical Centre. At the congress, the association officially created an Australasian Chapter. The council appointed Michael in his absence as interim president and the anaesthetist, Dr Chris Glynn, as secretary. Renowned neuroanatomist, Sir Sydney Sunderland, who was the first Australian to be an IASP councillor, agreed to be a co-founder and patron.[30]

Following Chris Glynn's return to Australia, he and Michael set to work. Sir Sydney Sunderland helped them create a draft constitution, which defined the organisation's goal: *To improve pain management by fostering pain research and education and developing clinical standards.* Sir Sydney Sunderland also promoted the new organisation to his network of pain professionals, attracting several Australian and New Zealand scientists and clinicians as founding members. In December 1978, Glynn, Sunderland and Michael Cousins invited eleven colleagues—anaesthetists, psychiatrists, neurosurgeons and pharmacologists—to serve on an interim committee. All were male and prominent in pain medicine. Five of them were anaesthetists, reflecting the pioneering role anaesthetists played in establishing pain clinics.[30]

John Bonica retired as the University of Washington's Chair of Anaesthesia in 1978. Disappointingly, with Bonica's departure, the funding he had attracted evaporated. Bonica's dominant personality and dogged persistence had ensured he secured sufficient funds to run the pain centre while he was there. After the University of Washington withdrew the pain centre's funding, Michael wrote a letter to its Vice-Chancellor, protesting the decision. 'He didn't even write back to me. So that was very, very sad, to see that wonderful facility, plus several top-class people, go into decline.' Through his interactions with John Bonica, Michael had internalised the professor's modus operandi. He set out to replicate it in Australia.

IASP's Australasian Chapter hosted its first annual scientific meeting, which Michael chaired, in May 1979 at Surfers Paradise in Queensland. Michael had organised it as a satellite to a combined conference for surgeons and anaesthetists, and to his amazement, it attracted 120 delegates. One of Michael's goals in arranging an integrated meeting was to improve communication between surgeons, anaesthetists and researchers to reduce the time it took for clinicians to adopt new treatments based on the results of the latest scientific studies. At the meeting, local and international pain experts shared their research findings in this rapidly growing field of medicine.[30]

Dr Bruce Rounsefell, who went on to head the pain management unit of Royal Adelaide Hospital for twenty-five years, took part in the meeting and was astonished to meet so many physicians treating people suffering from pain. 'It was a bit of a worldwide mini-explosion of sudden interest in pain,' he said. 'The mood in the room was electric, and everyone felt euphoric.'[31] The meeting attracted Professor Tony Yaksh from the Mayo Clinic in America as a keynote speaker. Yaksh, with his shaggy hair, bushy beard, moustache and tinted glasses thrilled the audience when he spoke about the use of local anaesthesia to block pain sensations in particular areas of the body. Capturing the exhilaration and optimism in pain medicine at the time, Yaksh said everyone in the pain world thought the ability to manage pain was close at hand.[30]

Sadly, later research revealed pain was far more complicated than anyone had imagined in those heady days.

6

THE RACE TO ADVANCE EPIDURAL PAIN RELIEF

IN the late 1970s, Michael and the Flinders team began a series of studies on epidural pain relief. A century earlier, during trials of epidural anaesthesia during labour, the Swiss obstetrician, Dr Oskar Kreis, had injected cocaine into the epidural space of six pregnant women. The lower part of the women's bodies were immediately anaesthetised, but they all suffered from severe nausea, vomiting and headache. This was the earliest report of the use of regional anaesthesia for the relief of labour pain.[32]

At the beginning of the twentieth century, the German gynaecologist, Dr Walter Stoeckel, repeated Kreis' procedure but replaced the cocaine with local anaesthetic. 'The result exceeded my expectations,' he wrote. 'The labour pains vanished, while the progress of labour remained unimpaired. The birth of the child followed so painlessly that the mother was totally unaware of it.'[33] In 1909 Stoeckel published a series of 141 case studies of epidural pain relief during labour.[34] Still, it wasn't until the 1960s that several researchers, such as Philip Bromage, started investigating epidural pain relief more comprehensively.

Throughout the 1970s, a team of researchers at the Mayo Clinic in the

United States investigated the effects of injecting morphine into the intrathecal space—the fluid-filled area between the innermost layer covering the spinal cord and the middle layer. They found it relieved the pain of several cancer patients. Professor Tony Yaksh led the team, and when he travelled to Australia in May 1979 for the Australasian Chapter's first scientific meeting, he visited Michael in Adelaide before heading north to the conference. The two researchers spent a full day discussing the latest developments in epidural pain relief.[35]

'Well, you must be able to inject morphine into the epidural space as well,' Michael suggested, 'because it would be much more valuable than injecting it into the intrathecal space. You could insert catheters into the epidural space and leave them there over a lengthy period.'

'I hadn't thought of that,' Yaksh said, 'but I'm not sure the opiates would get past the dura.[iii] Look, I'll tell you what. I'll give you a two-month start. You go ahead with it, and I won't do anything for two months. After that, I'm getting into it, too.'[15]

Yaksh's generosity surprised Michael. Scientists are usually highly competitive, and Michael had a strong competitive streak. After Yaksh's visit, the Flinders team kicked off a series of studies on epidural pain relief. In a break from the standard practice, they injected pethidine rather than a local anaesthetic into the epidural space. Michael and Mather rationalised that pethidine should be a more effective drug because, unlike other opioids, it had a mild local anaesthetic action in addition to its morphine-like pain relief properties.[27]

The first patient they tested with this technique was a middle-aged woman named Dora who suffered from severe lower back pain. Early one evening, Dora lay on a bed in the treatment room at the pain clinic where Michael had prepared her to receive an epidural injection. The nurses scurried around tidying up before they left for the day while Laurie Mather stood beside Dora's right shoulder chatting with her about what she was feeling. Two other researchers dressed in crisp white coats hovered at the end of the bed.[27]

Michael hooked up a thermometer to Dora's right big toe to measure any changes in her body temperature triggered by pethidine's local anaesthetic action. Then he injected pethidine into the epidural space in her back. After a few minutes, Michael asked Dora to describe her pain on a scale of one to ten.

'I don't have any pain,' she said.

'Do your legs feel numb?' Michael asked.

'No. They feel normal.'

Michael instructed Dora to wiggle her legs. She did.

These results astounded him because it meant the pethidine had not caused the loss of sensation or movement in the legs that occurred whenever he injected a local anaesthetic into a patient's epidural space. During the following weeks, Michael repeated the procedure on several more patients, and they experienced similar reactions. The Flinders team was ecstatic. An improved method of pain relief was seemingly within grasp![27]

Michael and his colleagues immediately wrote a letter describing the procedure and patients' responses. Then they faxed it to the British journal *The Lancet*, one of the world's oldest and best-known general medical journals. *The Lancet's* editor accepted the letter within twenty-four hours and published it in the following week's edition.[36] The letter suggested pain relief administered through the epidural space raised the possibility of 'selective spinal analgesia' because giving opioids avoided the loss of sensation and movement that usually accompanied the epidural administration of local anaesthetic.

This concept stimulated intense excitement around the world among researchers who were feverishly trying to find ways of delivering pain-relieving drugs via the epidural space.

'There was a bit of a race on between different research groups around the world to be the first to publish new methods of spinal pain relief,' Michael recalls. 'I think it happens every time something new and exciting appears on the horizon.'

It was an exhilarating time to be researching epidural pain relief. 'Our team became euphoric,' Michael said, adding that, at first, the team asked, 'Can it be true?' Then they became convinced it was right. He believes part of the reward of research is publishing and communicating the findings.

'It's a signal you've contributed to better understanding an illness, and it eggs you on to do more to see if you can improve the way we treat medical conditions.'

In August 1979, the Flinders team conducted a further clinical study with cancer patients undergoing chest surgery. They injected morphine into the epidural space during the operation and found the pain relief continued for several days after the surgery. This discovery delighted the researchers, but to their dismay, they noticed the breathing of two patients slowed and became shallow several hours after they had returned to the ward. Again, the team wrote to *The Lancet*, outlining their findings. The editor published the letter a few days later.[37] It was the first report of delayed depression of breathing associated with the injection of morphine into the epidural space.

The Flinders study on delayed respiratory depression was the start of a series by the team to determine how delayed respiratory depression occurred. The researchers realised morphine migrated slowly up the spinal cord; it took about three hours to travel to the brain, then more time to penetrate deep enough into the brain tissue to affect the breathing centre. This slow migration was why some patients experienced depressed breathing about ten or twelve hours after receiving the morphine.

During these hectic years of research and treating patients Michael continued to co-edit his textbook with Philip Bridenbaugh. They regularly liaised with the thirty-nine contributors but each of the authors was consumed by their day job, so it was a monumental challenge to ensure everyone submitted their chapters on time. Michael admits it took a mountain of tact, encouragement and pushing because each author was a leader in the field and extremely busy. But he said it was often worth the wait because the 'latest ones were those most worth waiting for'. Once the drafts arrived, Michael and Bridenbaugh edited the manuscripts. 'It was taxing but exhilarating,' Michael recalls.

Michael and Bridenbaugh finished their work on the manuscript in 1979, shortly before Michael's fortieth birthday, and J. B. Lippincott & Co. published the book in 1980.[38] It was the first comprehensive modern textbook on regional anaesthesia and pain. Many anaesthetists view *Neural Blockade in Clinical Anesthesia and Management of Pain*, now in its fourth edition, as the definitive book on regional anaesthesia and pain medicine.[29] Emeritus Professor Dan Carr, former Saltonstall Professor of Pain Research at Tufts University in Massachusetts, describes it as the 'desert island book' for anaesthetists on pain. 'If you were to find yourself on a desert island with only one book on pain, it is the one.'[39]

Several leading pain researchers claim the Flinders studies profoundly influenced the development of epidural pain relief in patients with acute, chronic and cancer pain.[21] Professor Allan Basbaum, Chair of Anatomy at the University of California, San Francisco, said the research 'is not only highly distinguished but without question has given rise to significant changes in the direction of research and practice of a newer generation of recognised scholars. It is not an understatement to say Professor Cousins' contributions were critical to the rapid adoption of these procedures in patients. His studies provided the evidence not only for utility and for defined safety limits but also established best practice procedures'.[40]

A few months after the Australasian Chapter's Surfers Paradise meeting, the International Association for the Study of Pain appointed Michael as treasurer. He felt honoured and welcomed the opportunity to deepen his relationships with IASP council members. 'I found it exhilarating to mix with the other council members, who were all first-rate pain researchers, because I heard firsthand about their latest discoveries. When I returned home, I brought this new knowledge to Australia, even before journals published it.' The opportunities he embraced energised him but combining his roles at Flinders University with IASP council responsibilities and writing textbooks, journal articles and reviews was taxing. He coped with his enormous workload by making a point of allocating two days to a project if he decided it was a priority. 'Because you won't get that time again, and it might decide yes or no for you.' He often advised his colleagues, 'Try not to take on more than you can reasonably handle,' but he routinely disobeyed his own rule.

The extra responsibilities Michael took on by building the Australian Pain Society and acting as IASP's treasurer left him feeling depleted. On summer nights after dinner, he relaxed by scooping leaves from the family's swimming pool. Highfield's garden was brimming with 150-year-old lemon-scented gum trees, oaks and elms, so keeping the pool free of leaves was an uphill battle. But Michael didn't mind; it calmed him and gave him time to ponder. He often thought about a book a colleague had lent him: the 1946 psychological memoir, *Man's Search for Meaning*, by Viktor Frankl, a Viennese neurologist and psychiatrist who had survived Auschwitz.[41] Frankl chronicled his experiences as a prisoner during the Second World War and shared his insights into how to persevere during the toughest times. He maintained the secret to spiritual survival lies in finding a purpose and taking responsibility for ourselves and other human beings. He believed we are only able to make the world a better place when we are confident of the aim motivating us. Frankl's message resonated with Michael. 'I think it includes ideas important to pain and to anyone who wants to live a meaningful life.' It reinforced his mission to improve the treatment of pain.

In late August 1980, Michele's parents visited the Cousins for the school holidays. Michele, Poppy, Trenham and the three boys drove six hours north of Adelaide to the Flinders Ranges. They stayed at Parachilna Gorge for five days and on the way home fell in love with Wilpena Pound, an elliptical crown of serrated mountains with a sunken natural amphitheatre in its centre. They stopped to walk up Wilpena. Poppy and Richard said they felt unwell. Poppy remained in the car with Jonathan, but despite feeling off-colour, Richard joined his mother, grandfather and James on a walk. Afterwards they returned to Adelaide and enjoyed a quiet Sunday night at home, unaware of what lay ahead for them.

The next morning Poppy felt ill with flu, collapsed on the bathroom floor and hit her head. She needed stitches, so Michael took her to Flinders Medical Centre and the doctors admitted her to a medical ward. Poppy's condition started to improve but later on Wednesday morning, Richard had a fever and vomited several times. The family's general practitioner was unable to do a home visit, so Michele carried her son downstairs, bundled him into the back seat of the car and drove him to the doctor's surgery. As soon as the GP felt Richard's racing pulse, he told Michele her son was critically ill, and she should rush him to Adelaide Children's Hospital. The paediatrician tried every known treatment to save the eight-year-old, but the virus had overwhelmed his heart muscle. Tragically, Richard died the same day of viral myocarditis.

Michael was engulfed by grief, and he struggled to take in Richard's death. He felt a searing guilt that he had been working rather than at home to care for his beloved son. Geoff Cousins flew to Adelaide as soon as he heard about Richard, and he helped Michael and Michele organise their son's funeral. He also tried to keep James and Jonathan busy. Michael was so distraught that Geoff worried his brother would never recover from Richard's death.

Geoff Cousins credits Michele with being a tower of strength for Michael and the entire family after Richard died.[42] Michele felt she had no other choice. 'I couldn't afford to collapse in a heap. I had to look after Mum after she returned home from hospital, and James and Jonathan needed me to keep their lives going.'[5]

One thing that helped the couple deal with their grief was prayer. In the years following Richard's illness and death, Michael and Michele talked lovingly about him with their children. While Michael found it difficult to talk about Richard, Michele openly spoke about what had happened. She was determined to let other parents know about the risk of viral myocarditis when their children have the flu and need to take care.

After Richard died, Michele soon became pregnant. She and Michael were thrilled to discover they were having twins. A week before the twins were due, the obstetrician decided to induce them. Michele was delighted that obstetric anaesthetist, Dr Peter Brownridge, gave her an epidural. Brownridge wrote an acclaimed textbook on pain relief options during labour and Michele felt in wise hands.

After a long labour, the first baby, a boy, safely arrived. Michele caught a glimpse of him during the delivery. 'Oh my gosh,' she thought, 'he looks exactly the same as Richard and Michael'. However, the second baby was stuck in a breech position and suffering fetal distress. The obstetrician told Michele she needed an emergency caesarian. Michele wanted to see her baby being born and asked Brownridge whether he could just 'top up the epidural'.[5] But he shook his head, insisting he give her a general anaesthetic. One hour and two minutes later, a healthy baby girl arrived. It was nine months and two weeks after Richard had died. Michele and Michael were ecstatic and named the twins Jane and Christopher. They viewed the newborns as a special gift and felt immensely blessed after losing Richard.

Meanwhile, the epidural analgesia studies catapulted the Flinders team onto the world stage in pain medicine research. Michael felt elated and thought his efforts to overcome what had seemed like insurmountable obstacles had finally paid off. Shortly after *The Lancet* letters appeared, the journal *Anesthesiology* invited Michael and Laurie Mather to co-author a comprehensive review of the science of spinal opioids.[43] Michael is proud of the review, which is seminal in the field of epidural anaesthesia and analgesia.[44] As well as co-writing this review, Michael accepted invitations to write journal articles, reviews, editorials and chapters for textbooks on pain.

Michael worried that the Flinders pain management team didn't have a simple system in place in the surgical wards to provide continuous pain relief for patients after an operation. He wanted patients to be able to adjust the amount of medication they received according to their pain level. In late 1980, the team set to work to develop an implantable system, adapting an existing system that delivered a constant flow of cancer drugs to patients via the epidural space. During the following months, they engineered a device, then studied the effectiveness of different opioids delivered by this implanted system. These patient-controlled devices enabled hospital patients to fine-tune the quantity of pain-relieving drugs they received intravenously by pressing a button. An important feature was an inbuilt safeguard to prevent overdose.[45]

IASP's Australasian Chapter held its third scientific meeting at Flinders University in 1981. Michael was determined to keep the meeting low-priced, so the Flinders' team created the books of abstracts by photocopying and hand binding them.[30] John Liebeskind, a psychologist and neuroscientist from the University of California in Los Angeles, presented the first scientific paper. He stood at the podium in the echoey lecture theatre, checking his notes while the delegates noisily filed in and found a seat. The room was alive with excited chatter, and a sense of expectation hung in the air. Michael sat at the front of the theatre admiring

Liebeskind's 'distinctive look'. His hair had turned a silvery grey earlier than usual and he had a baby face. Michael thought Liebeskind exuded warmth and he knew from colleagues the psychologist was famous for his bonhomie and love of the heuristic. Liebeskind held a thick bundle of typed A4 pages. When Michael noticed the bulkiness of the speech and lack of overhead projector slides, he dreaded an hour of listening to a presentation read from a script.

'But once John Liebeskind started speaking, he eloquently painted a picture of the field of pain medicine at that moment in time,' Michael recalls. 'He entranced and inspired everyone in the room. I sat transfixed.'

Another pain medicine researcher who inspired Michael was Dr John Loeser, the University of Washington's Professor of Neurological Surgery. In 1982 the University of Washington appointed Loeser as Director of its Multidisciplinary Pain Center and he set out to rebuild the pain centre to its former glory. Loeser worked closely with the psychologist, Dr Bill Fordyce. Shortly after Loeser began his new role, he and Fordyce were overjoyed to discover an empty ward at the university's hospital. They were even more elated when the hospital administrators allowed the pair to convert the ward into facilities for people being treated for chronic pain. Using this specialist space, the two researchers created a structured three-week inpatient pain management program.[46]

Loeser and Fordyce based the structured program on an approach to dealing with chronic pain that was innovative at the time—behavioural psychology—using social reinforcers to change abnormal behaviours. In the case of patients with chronic pain, this meant encouraging them to gradually increase their level of activity and at the same time tapering the amount of medication they used. Michael read several journal articles by Loeser and Fordyce. He wanted to learn more about behavioural psychology and the structured program, so he planned a visit to the University of Washington.

Sadly, this trip was soon relegated to the backburner when Michael received a panicked phone call from his mother Marjorie. She told him Hedley had suffered a stroke and an ambulance had rushed him to Royal North Shore Hospital. In shock and feeling as if he was on autopilot,

Michael drove to Adelaide airport and caught the next flight to Sydney.

When he reached the hospital Michael ran up the stairs two at a time to his father's ward. What he saw deeply distressed him. His father's face was ashen, and he couldn't speak, something that Michael knew would frustrate Hedley because he was such a consummate communicator. Michael, his siblings and Marjorie kept a vigil by Hedley's bedside for five days. But on the fifth day Hedley suffered a second stroke and died. Michael loved, admired and respected his father and was distraught to lose him. He also worried about his mother and how she would cope.

Several months after Hedley's death, Michael travelled to Seattle for an IASP meeting. While there, he visited John Loeser at the University of Washington's pain centre. Loeser told him that most patients at the pain clinic had experienced daily pain for longer than three months. Like the patients Michael saw at Flinders Medical Centre, the patients' diagnoses rarely explained the severity of their pain, disability and depression or heavy use of medications. Loeser, who was 'larger than life' according to Michael, told his visitor in his characteristic 'big' warm voice, that in the years leading up to their referral to the clinic, many patients were like a billiard ball caroming off one cushion to the other—as each physician referred them to another physician. These patients took multiple opioids from different prescribers and, despite using strong analgesics, still complained of unrelenting pain. Michael nodded, knowing his patients too depended on opioids that didn't relieve their pain. 'That's why we try to help patients realise opioids may not be helping them,' Loeser said. 'As you and I both know, opioids can sensitise pain receptors, flaring up the pain.'

He explained that one of the university pain team's top priorities was to help patients gradually reduce and discontinue their use of opioids. 'Their pain doesn't get any worse and often decreases, much to the patients' surprise,' he added.

Michael's visit to the University of Washington impressed on him the urgent need to ramp up the interdisciplinary pain services at Flinders. He returned to Adelaide more determined than ever to access the funding he required to do this.

7

THE POWER OF RELATIONSHIPS

JOHN Bonica had taught Michael the critical importance of educating politicians and bureaucrats about the costs of unrelieved pain. Michael tried to influence federal and state-based decision-makers, but his skills were as a doctor rather than a lobbyist. He had observed his parents and uncles advocate for change, and dipped his big toe in the water as a university student and registrar. But during his first five years at Flinders, he felt frustrated that he made little progress in making pain management a political issue or government priority. It deeply disappointed him.

These days, media relations and advocacy training are more commonplace for people in senior positions, but back then, many organisations didn't provide such training. Instead, Michael learned on the job, gaining skills through trial and error. A further difficulty was that most advocacy in Adelaide occurred through personal relationships formed at school and university. As a Sydneysider trying to influence South Australia's politicians and bureaucrats, Michael was at a slight disadvantage.

South Australia's progressive Labor Government supported the use of heroin for pain relief in patients with terminal cancer despite repeated studies failing to support heroin's effectiveness. It was a 'political hot potato'. In the early 1980s, South Australia's Health Minister, the veterinarian John Cornwall, telephoned Michael to discuss the heroin issue. Cornwall was a reformer and advocated for citizens to have more control over their health so they could take action themselves to improve it.[47] When he phoned, Michael was at home recovering from surgery for surfer's ear, a condition in which the ear canal narrows so much it is difficult to hear. The surgeon said it was the worst case of surfer's ear he had ever seen. Michael developed the painful condition after decades of bodysurfing and collecting grains of sand in his ears. For eighteen months preceding the surgery, every night when he put his head on his pillow, Michael could hear his heartbeat because of the pressure inside his ears, which was annoying and stopped him from falling asleep.

When Michele visited Michael in hospital, she thought 'they've taken half his brain away' because one side of his face and head were painted bright yellow.[5] The surgery left Michael with tinnitus, which is ringing in the ears or noises such as hissing, whooshing or buzzing. Because he felt so unwell, his initial reaction to Cornwall's phone call was to tell the minister to 'jump in the lake'. But Cornwall asked Michael to lead a study on whether heroin relieved severe cancer pain. Michael thought back to John Bonica's advice about nurturing supporters within political ranks. Instead of rebuffing Cornwall, he suggested they meet at Flinders Medical Centre. Cornwall agreed. Before ending the call, Michael added, 'Look, if you really feel we should pursue this, I'll do my best to get people involved, but I can't promise anything'.

A few weeks later, John Cornwall was due at Flinders for the meeting. Michael anxiously waited at the pain clinic's front entrance for him, worrying the Minister might cancel at the last minute if an urgent issue cropped up at Parliament House. Michael bore the weight of the pain team's expectations on his shoulders, and felt it deeply. As he waited, he rehearsed in his head what he planned to say to Cornwall. Suddenly, out of the corner of his eye, he spotted a white government car inching along the university driveway. The late-model Holden pulled up in front of the pain clinic, and the Minister alighted. The minister's two male staff flanked him. Michael led them into the pain clinic, introduced them to several team members, then showed the trio the pain centre's facilities. The ministerial advisers walked behind Michael and Cornwall, scribbling notes in small pocketbooks. During the tour, a hushed silence filled the pain centre. The atmosphere was tense with anticipation.

By the time the delegation reached Michael's office, a bone china tea set was waiting for them on the low coffee table. Michael offered his guests a cup of tea, and while pouring it, he chatted with Cornwall. He handed around the tea and offered everyone a wholemeal cookie that Michele had baked the previous day. Teacups rattled on their saucers while Michael told Cornwall about the two pain clinic patients he had invited to the meeting. One, a woman in her fifties, struggled with cancer pain, and the other, a man in his forties, suffered from chronic lower back pain after a workplace injury.

Once Michael's guests finished their tea, the two patients filed in, shook hands with Cornwall, then sat on the black sofa. The woman fidgeted, crossing and uncrossing her legs. Michael invited the pair to tell the minister about their treatment regimen at the pain clinic. Neither patient had used heroin. The man hesitated, then described in minute detail how his exercise program and counselling had helped him to manage his pain. The woman joined in the conversation, explaining how an epidural morphine pump had settled her unrelenting pain.

Cornwall asked the patients several questions, then praised them for sharing their stories with him so honestly. After the patients departed, Cornwall looked across at Michael. 'I'm getting the feeling this heroin business is a bit of a distraction,' he admitted. 'The actual issue is we're not applying what we know about the treatment of pain.'

One week later, Cornwall's wife, Patrice, made an appointment to see Michael. When she arrived at the pain clinic for her consultation, Michael could see by her stiff walk and sagging shoulders that she was in severe pain.

'I've had lower back pain for years,' she said, grimacing. 'I've tried everything. Nothing's helped.'

Michael asked Patrice a series of questions about her condition, then examined her. Afterwards, he told her that her original back injury had transitioned to chronic back pain.

'Sadly, it's impossible to cure chronic pain because it's a malfunction in the way your nervous system processes pain signals,' he explained, 'but I can help you better manage your pain, so it doesn't affect your life so much'.

Patrice returned a few weeks later after starting a daily program of stretches and gentle strengthening exercises. She had also seen the pain clinic psychologist. Michael asked how she was feeling.

Patrice beamed. 'I'm much better thank you. I'm thrilled.'

During the following few weeks, Michael and John Cornwall met several times to discuss Michael's funding needs. They got along well, possibly because both were ardent reformers. 'We saw eye to eye,' Michael recalls. 'We both wanted to improve health care.' A few months later, South Australia's Health Department granted the Flinders pain centre four years of funding—enough to build a purpose-designed interdisciplinary pain management facility with consulting rooms, an operating theatre and treatment rooms. Michael also secured ongoing funding to recruit research and clinical staff. Finally, he felt as if he was making some headway. But it wasn't all plain sailing because the hospital's administrators tried to siphon off some of the funds for other projects they considered more worthy.

'I had to push hard to get the senior hospital administrators to give me the funds,' Michael said. 'One of them told me there was no money in the allocation for cleaners and that without funding for them, I couldn't expand the pain clinic or appoint anyone new to the team.'

Michael worried that most politicians didn't recognise the personal and societal costs of untreated pain, so in 1982 he invited Michael MacKellar, the then Federal Health Minister, to open the IASP Australasian Chapter's fourth scientific meeting. He aimed to increase awareness among politicians of the costs of chronic pain. Two years later, the Chapter commissioned the health economist, Paul Gross, to undertake a pilot study on the cost of chronic pain to provide the evidence needed to educate government officials and encourage them to increase funding for pain research and treatment. That year the Australasian Chapter also shortened its name to the Australian Pain Society.[30]

In 1983 Professor Dominick P. Purpura, Stanford University's Dean of Medicine, wrote to Michael, inviting him to apply to be the medical school's head of anaesthesia. Purpura also approached San Francisco-based Professor Ron Miller, a pioneer in anaesthesia research. Michael was uncertain about moving his family to America, but the opportunity exhilarated him. He set to work, meticulously preparing a proposal outlining his research achievements and publications. He bound it in a vivid red cover and carried it with him to San Francisco. At Stanford, Purpura told Michael the anaesthesia department's budget was US$1 million each year. Michael was astonished. This was a sizeable amount at the time and would enable him to fund a comprehensive pain research program. As part of the interview process, Michael delivered a lecture to an assembled panel of professors on the value he would bring to Stanford University.

Afterwards, he had one-to-one meetings with several Stanford professors to gain their support for his appointment. Once he had completed the interview process, he flew back to Adelaide. During the flight home, he reflected on his performance and beat himself up for all the things he forgot to say. Still, he felt pleased with the feedback he had received from the Stanford professors.

To his immense surprise, within two weeks, Michael received a faxed letter from Purpura offering him the position. In two minds about leaving Australia, Michael and Michele, 'paced the bedroom floor for several nights agonising over the pros and cons' of uprooting their children. Michael worried about his mother and wanted to live close to her in case she needed help. Michele felt the same way about her elderly parents. The couple was also keen for their children to grow up in Australia. Still, Michael knew it would be far more challenging to build a pain centre of international standing in Adelaide than at Stanford.

As he wrestled with this decision, a friend from Stanford faxed him a newspaper article announcing Dominick Purpura had retired. Michael suspected 'all bets would be off'; a new dean would not necessarily honour the financial commitments Purpura had made. Based on this latest news and his misgivings about moving to America, Michael decided against taking up the role at Stanford. Instead, following John Bonica's advice to 'never, never give up,' he settled on persevering despite the resource constraints and bureaucratic struggles he faced each day at Flinders.

In 1984 Michael and Michele flew to Seattle for an IASP world congress. Michele joined her husband on the trip because IASP intended to appoint Michael as its Vice-President at the congress. And the couple wanted to celebrate Michele's fortieth birthday in a memorable way. Michael felt honoured to take on the role of Vice-President, especially because it meant he would work alongside Ronald Melzack, who was the association's president.

Working with Ronald Melzack in his new role reinforced Michael's commitment to doing everything in his power to advance the field of pain medicine. The two researchers developed a great rapport, and Michael soon discovered they were both thinking along similar lines about the organisation's future focus. During this period, Michael promoted his idea for the association to increase its focus on acute and cancer pain because it had focused on chronic pain since its inception in 1973. Several scientists from among the membership opposed this proposal, but Melzack supported it, and so did influential council member Kathleen Foley. To 'move things along,' Melzack and Michael set up a task force on acute pain management chaired by Dr Brian Ready from Seattle. The task force quickly got to work creating a manual on the treatment of acute pain that, once completed, would help the association become recognised as an authority on acute pain. It also helped IASP to attract pain researchers and clinicians to congresses where they could learn about the explosion of knowledge in pain diagnosis, prevention and treatment.

Another issue Melzack and Michael tackled was promoting international interaction and expanding the association's membership. The pair wanted the organisation to be more inclusive of professionals from developing countries and nations with currency difficulties. But some council members were unsympathetic. 'If they can't pay the fees, they can't be members,' a few detractors argued. This attitude deeply disappointed

Michael, and he insisted all pain professionals had an equal right to join the organisation. Michael and Melzack worked out a more inclusive approach. But it took years to put in place. It wasn't until a meeting stretching late into the night in the Seattle home of one of the council's members that they finally 'hammered out a strategy'.[15]

An ambitious project Michael instigated in the mid-1980s was setting up the International Pain Foundation to raise funds for pain research. The idea came to him in the plane en route to an IASP council meeting in Buenos Aires, Argentina. Scribbling notes on the back of his agenda papers during the flight, he asked an assistant to type them up as soon as he arrived at the meeting. He tried to distribute the notes to the council, but some members protested. They were not keen on discussing the idea because it wasn't on the meeting's agenda and information about it was not in the council papers. Michael couldn't distribute the notes, but he 'managed to say some words about it, planting the seeds'. By a stroke of good luck, the influential council member, John Liebeskind, had also been contemplating the notion of having a separate fundraising body. But at the time, only he and Michael supported it. 'John Liebeskind set the wheels in motion,' Michael said, 'and we both pushed it forward, but it was an uphill battle.' Liebeskind continued to lobby his council colleagues, and gradually built a coalition of support. He also convinced the fresh orange juice magnate and philanthropist, Robert Wald, to provide seed funding of US$250,000 to kickstart the foundation.[15]

Around the same time, the journal *Pain* accepted the Flinders research on the delivery of opioids via the epidural space in patients with chronic pain.[48] Michael was elated because he felt it recognised the Flinders team's research prominence. Another pleasing development was that Australia's National Health and Medical Research Council set up a working group charged with developing clinical guidelines for severe pain. 'Long overdue,' according to Michael. The research council invited Michael to take part in the working group that included several distinguished Australian pain medicine professionals. The council's chair asked the working group to base the guidelines on the latest research to improve community and government awareness of severe pain and the urgent need for advancements in pain research, treatment and education. Michael was relieved to see this development and hoped it would convince governments around the nation to fund improved pain assessment and treatment. But the extra workload kept Michael locked up in his study on weekends. He knew he was hiding away in the basement study too often but felt fortunate he could take work home. It meant he could combine writing with spending time with Michele and his children.

By the mid-1980s, the Flinders pain team had attracted substantial media interest, helping to raise awareness of pain management, particularly chronic and cancer pain. In August 1985, the *Weekend Australian* published a feature story on some of the techniques the team had developed.[49] The article explained that the group's most unique method was injecting painkilling drugs directly into the epidural space via a tiny catheter attached to a pump.[50] The journalist, Louise Boylen, described the technique in minute detail, aiming to de-mystify it. She said the morphine pump enabled cancer patients to remain mobile and out of hospital because community nurses could top up the catheter in the comfort of a patient's home.[51] By the time News Limited published the article, the Flinders team had successfully treated two hundred patients with the morphine pump, and Michael hoped the publicity would mean he would treat many more people in the same way. However, given the pain clinic's limited resources, he knew this would put it under immense pressure. Still, he persisted, determined to help as many patients as possible, passionately believing pain management was a fundamental human right.

Although Michael was willing to 'ruffle a few feathers' within the anaesthesia profession, he always veered on the side of diplomacy. He modelled his behaviour on that of his father, whom he considered a 'true gentleman'. Harnessing every opportunity to urge his colleagues to improve the standard of pain management in Australia, in 1986 he wrote to Dr Ross Holland, Dean of the Faculty of Anaesthetists within the Royal Australasian College of Surgeons.[52] In his letter, he noted that the anaesthesia profession had been slow to embrace pain research, teaching and treatment. He also lamented the lack of resources dedicated to pain medicine. Describing the explosive growth in new knowledge, he declared

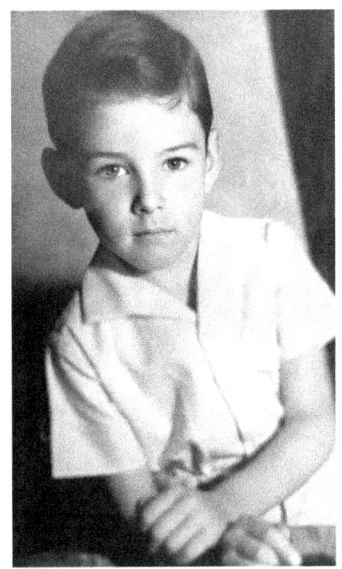
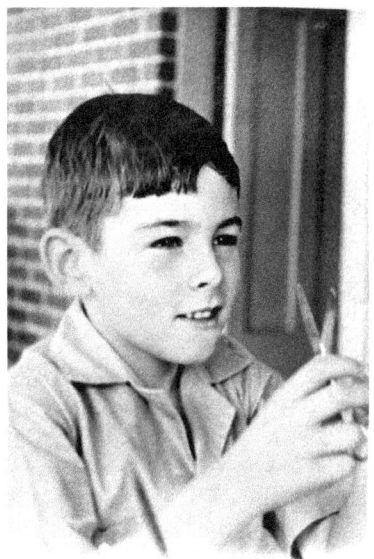

Michael as a young boy.

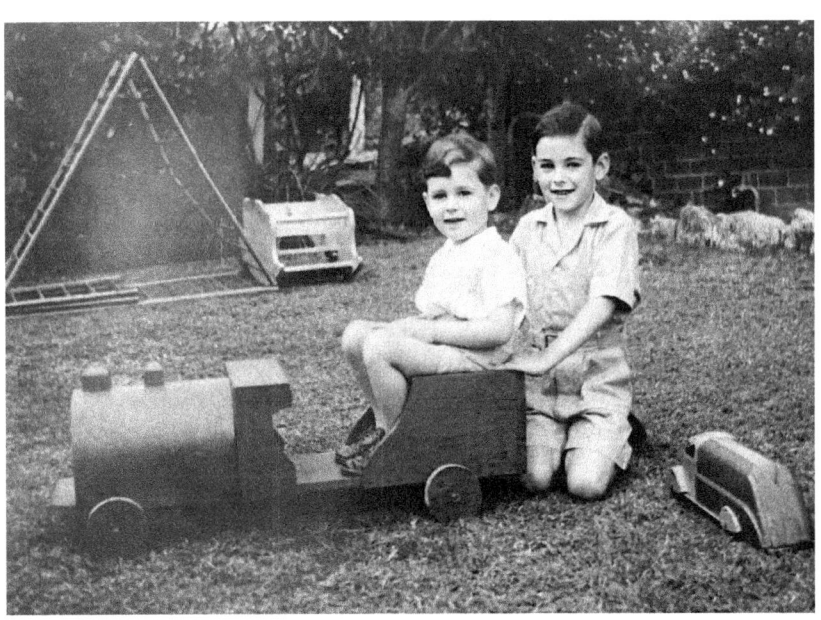

Geoff and Michael Cousins.

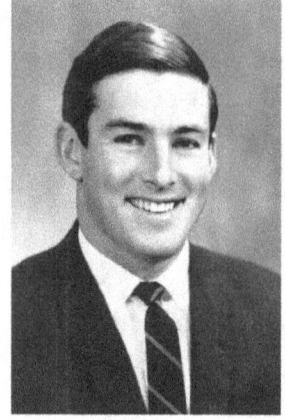

MICHAEL JOHN COUSINS

At Shore School, Mike was academically successful, a good sportsman and a high principled senior prefect.
He is still a "good sport".
Mike is well known—
To the tutors and professors, as a keen student and earnest, diplomatic student representative.
To all the students, who repeatedly voted him Year-Representative, as an optimistic, affable leader and as organizer of the memorable (and subsequently banned) Second and Third Year Dinners.
To his friends, as a vigorous and successfully competitive athlete, footballer, squash-player, skier, car-driver, humorist and "life-of-the-party".
To his critics, as a bad poet and hut-wrecker with a poor tolerance to Ethanol.
To the nurses.
Personality, plausibility and sincerity ensure his success.

Sydney University Medical School Year Book, 1961.

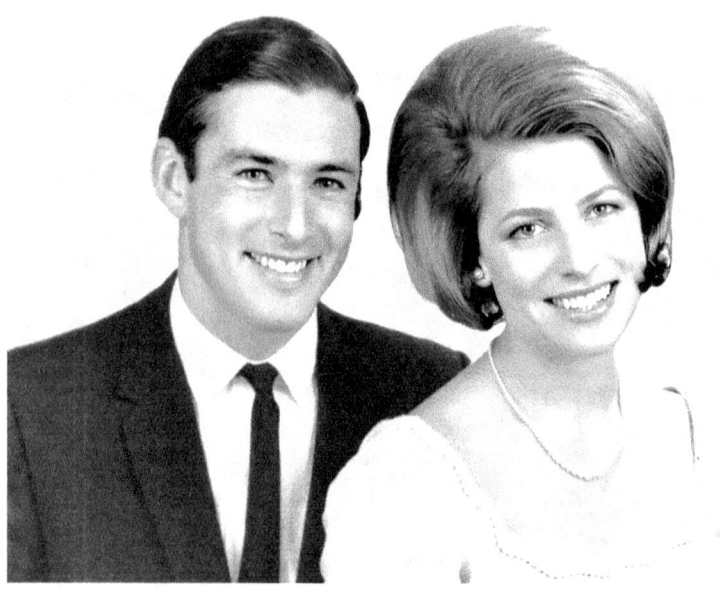

Michael and his fiancee, Michele Old, March 1967.

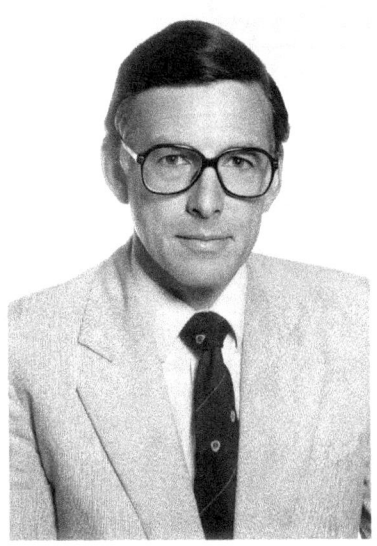
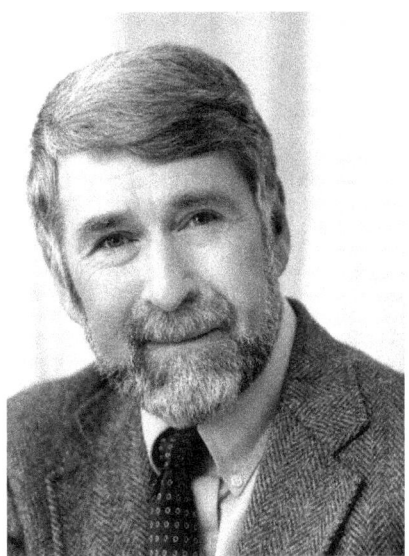

Michael, 1988.   Laurie Mather, 1991.

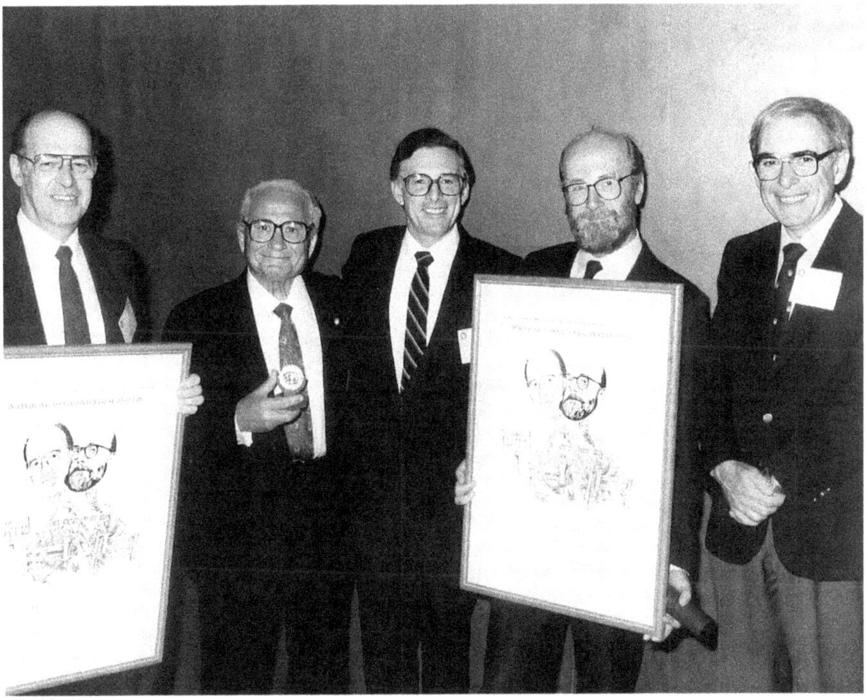

L to R: Ronald Melzack, John Bonica, Michael,
Patrick Wall, Issy Pilowsky, 1990.

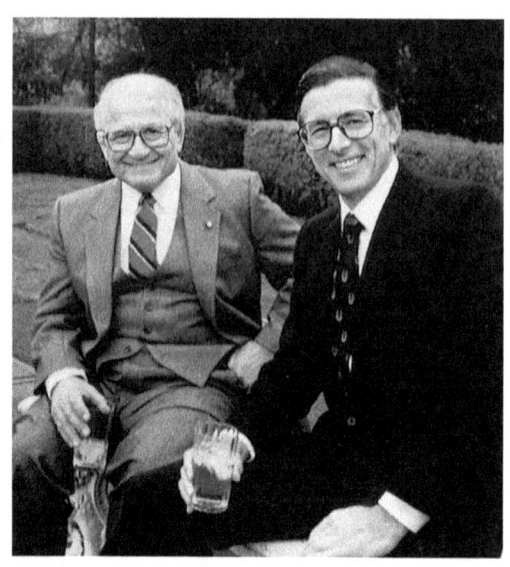

John Bonica and Michael in Seattle, April 1987.

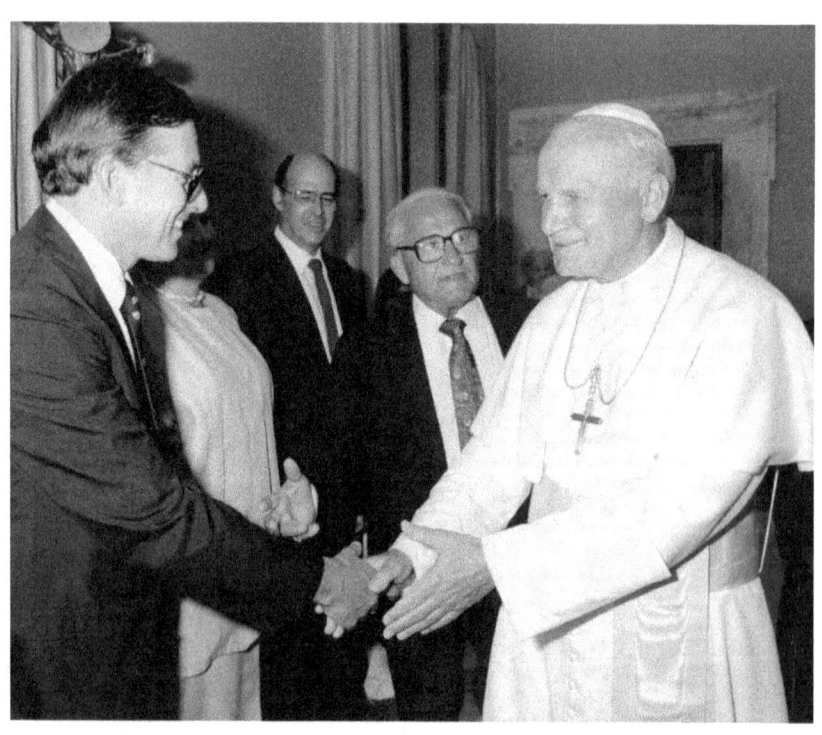

Michael, Lucy Melzack, Ronald Melzack, John Bonica with
Pope John Paul II, 1987.

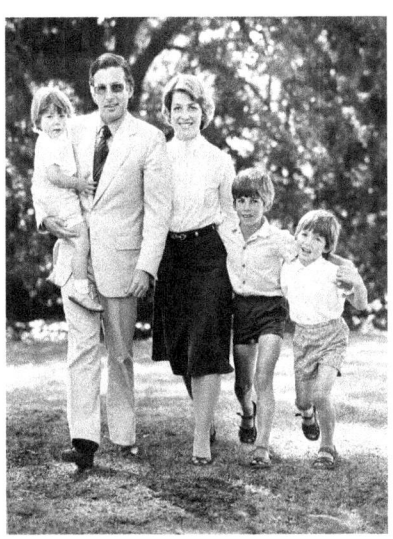

L to R: Jonathan, James and
Richard Cousins, 1976
(Photo: David Simpson).

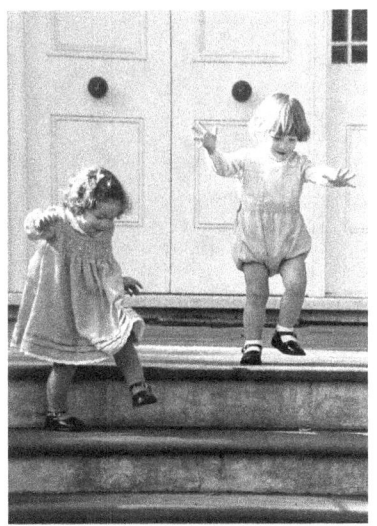

Jane and Chris Cousins
aged 2
(Photo: David Simpson).

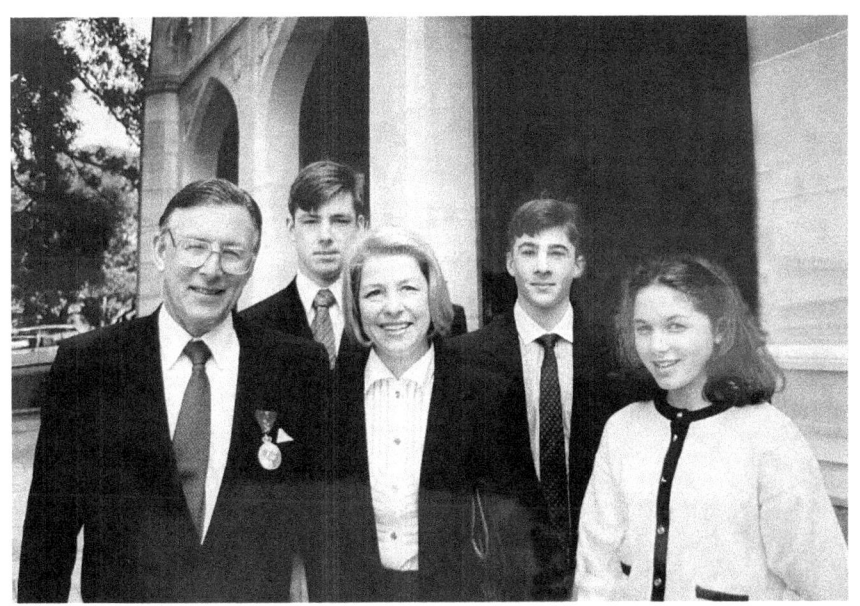

Michael, Jonathan, Michele, Chris and Jane,
Government House, 1994.

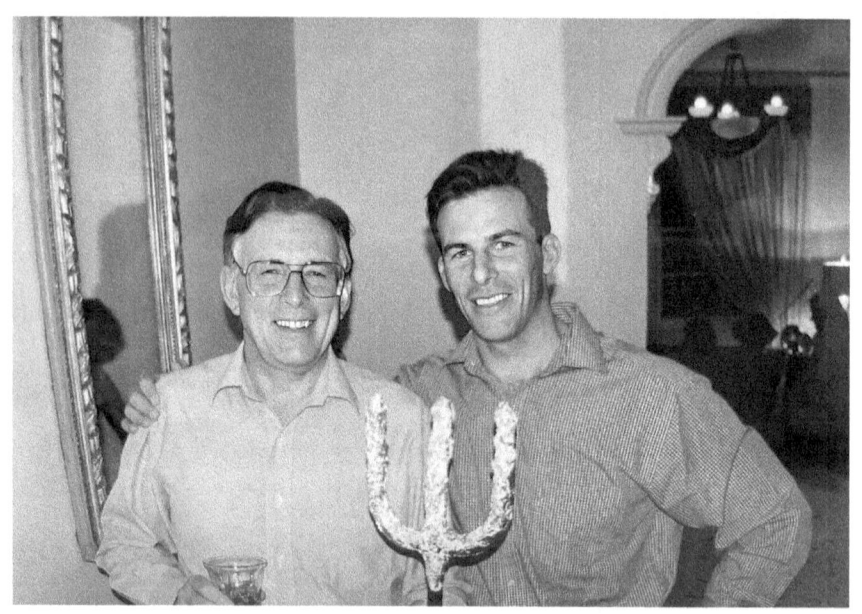

Michael and James Cousins at Michael's 60th birthday party, November 1999.

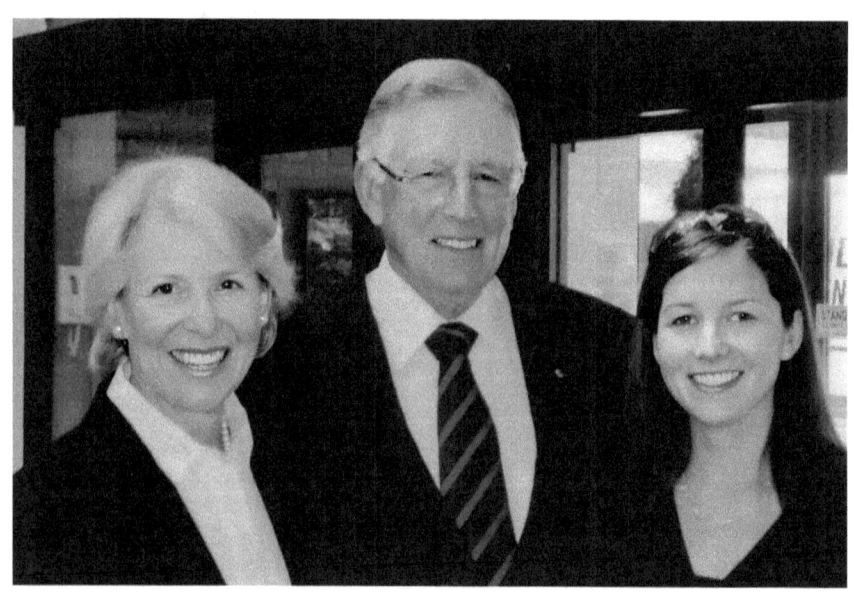

Michele, Michael and Jane Kuehn (nee Cousins), Ontario.

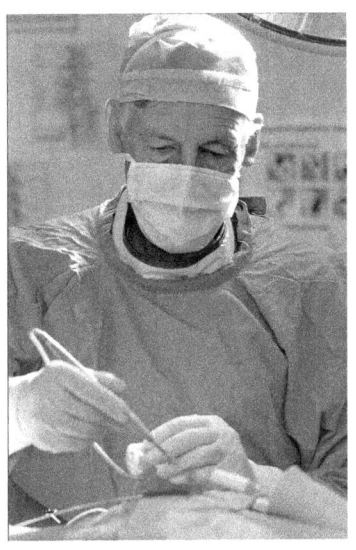

Michael during a pain management procedure.

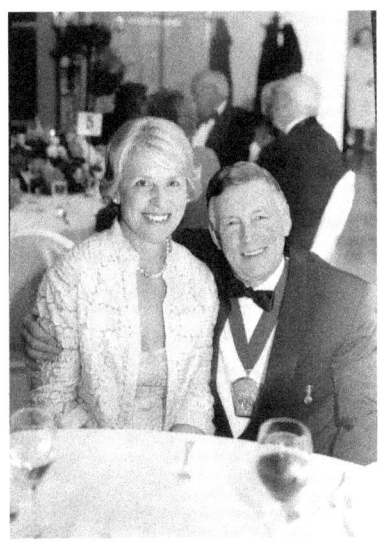

Michele and Michael, Melbourne, June 2006.

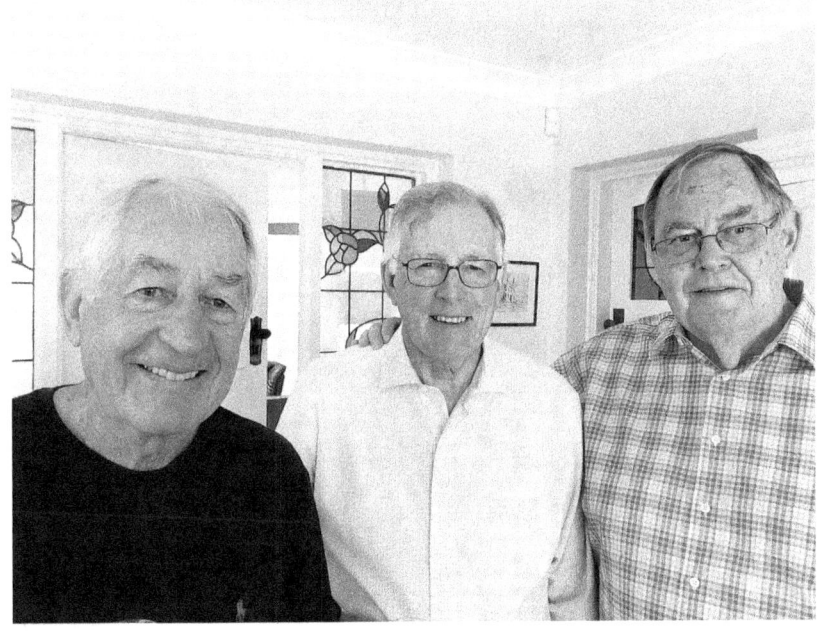

Michael with childhood friends Fergus Munro and Ray Chapman.

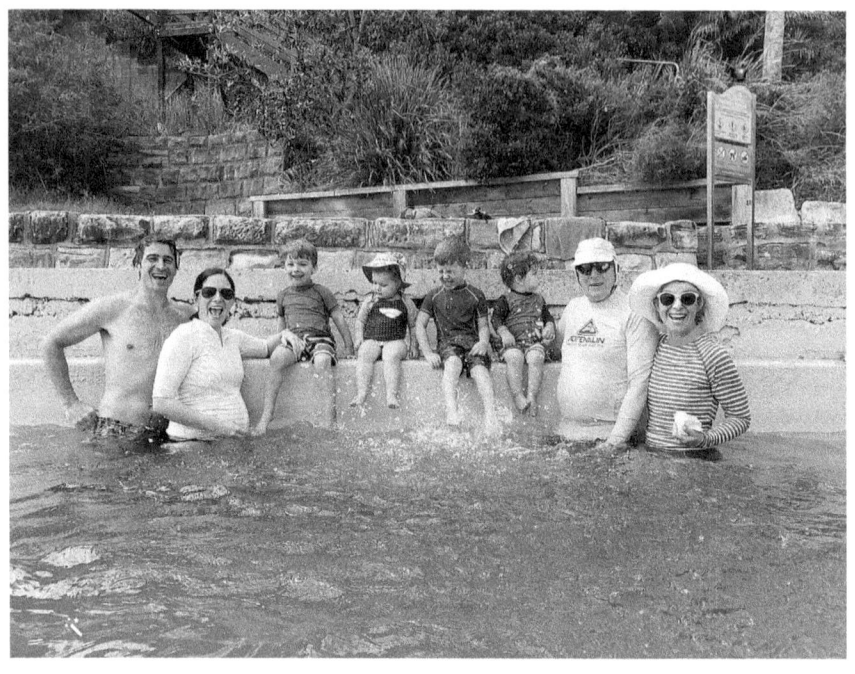

L to R: Chris Cousins, Jane Kuehn, Max, Mila, Henry, Rich, Michael and Michele, 2017.

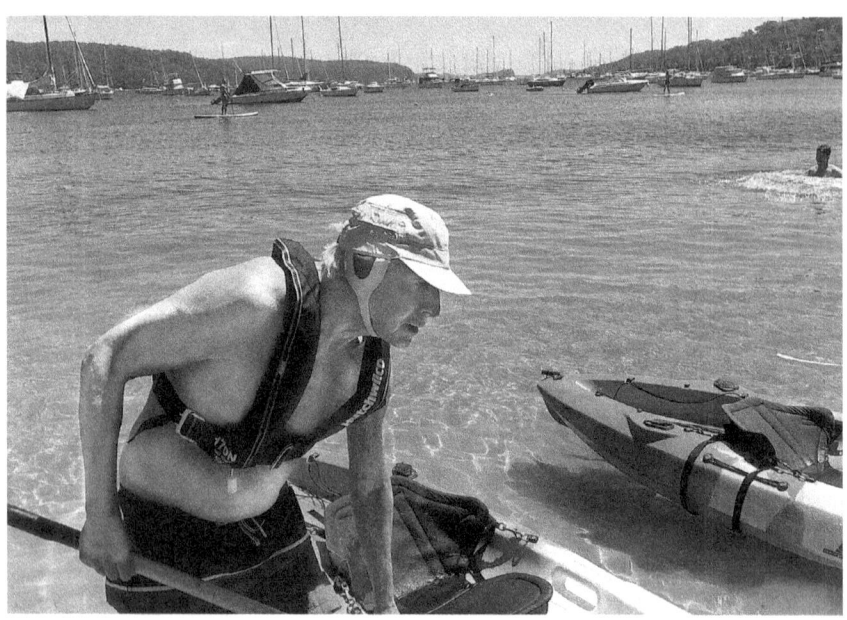

Michael paddling at Pittwater, January 2021.

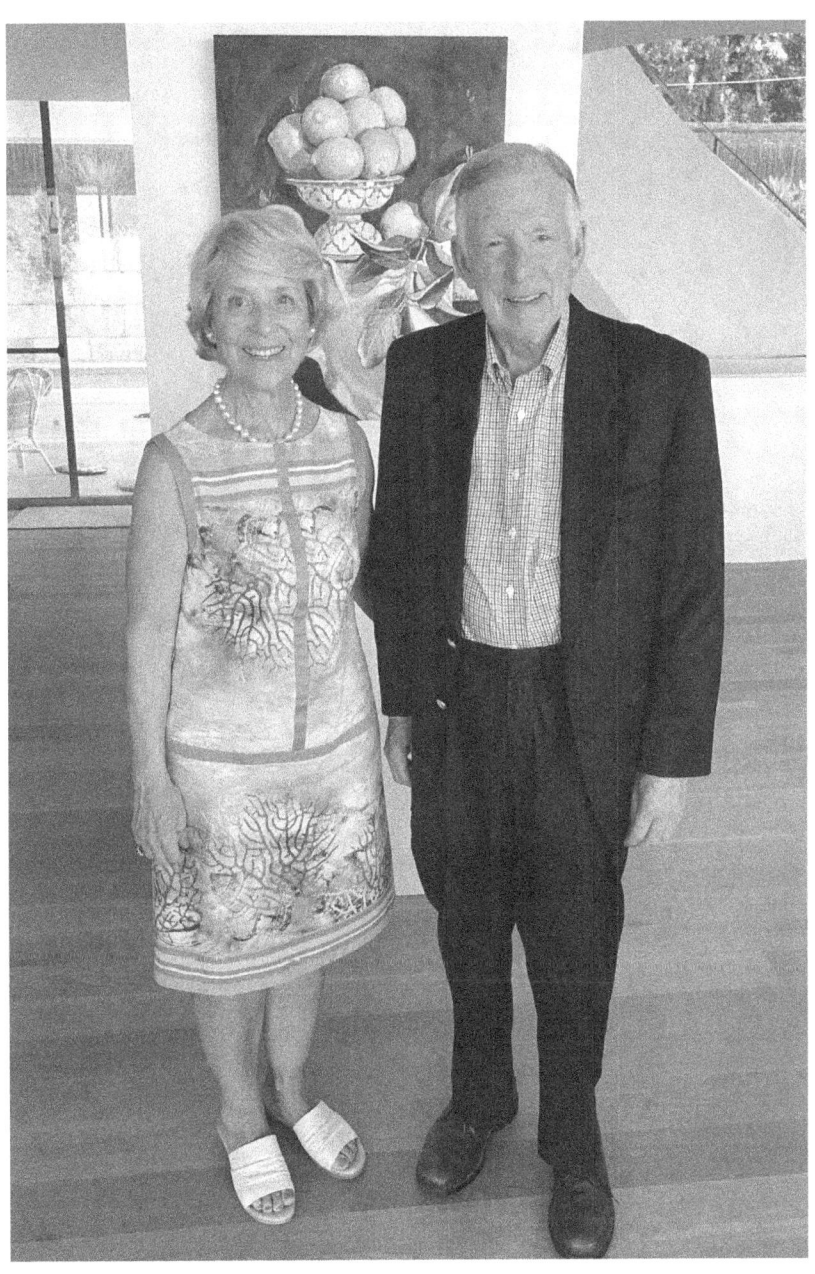

Michele and Michael, 2021.

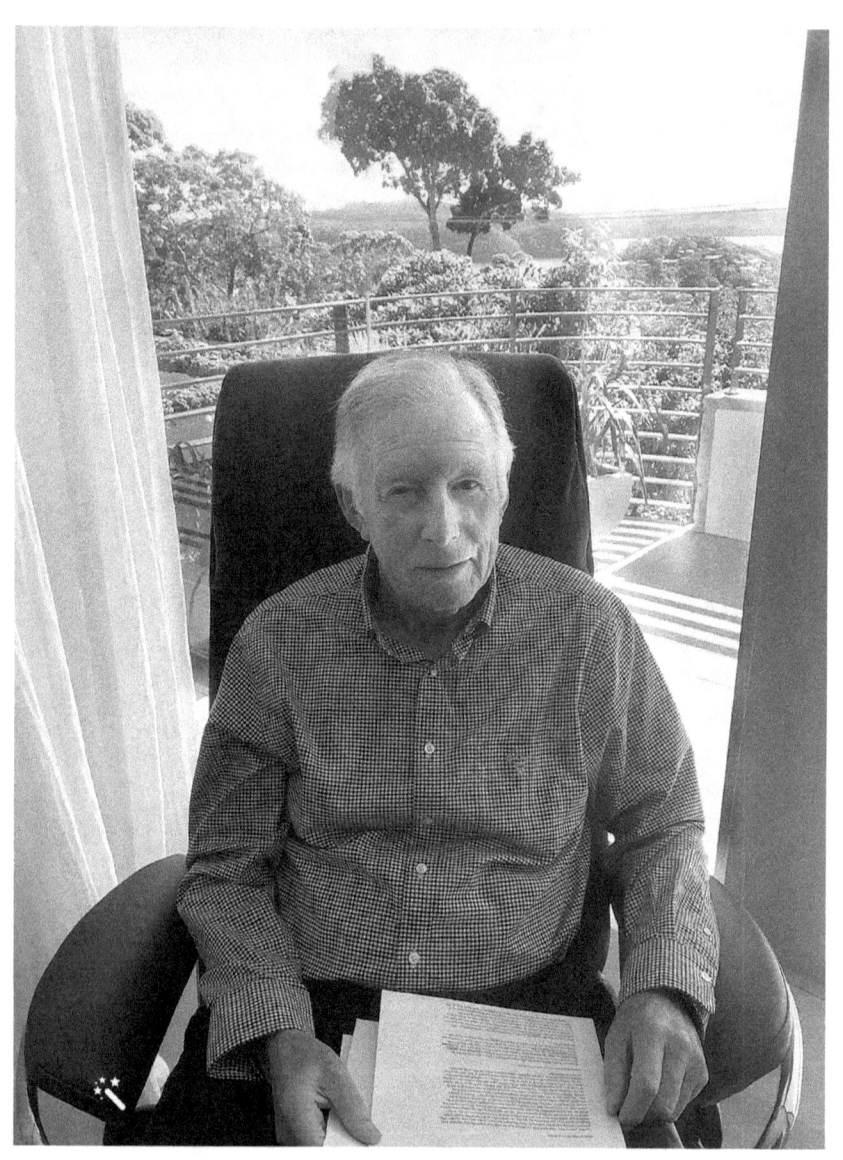

Michael reading this book's manuscript, 2021.

that the treatment of both acute and chronic pain was emerging as one of the most important and exciting challenges of modern medicine. Exhorting the Faculty of Anaesthetists to embrace pain management, he wrote: 'Pain management units should be an important and substantial part of every department of anaesthesia and intensive care in the major hospitals in the country. These units should provide clinical care in both acute and chronic pain. They should play an important part in undergraduate and postgraduate teaching and support research.'[52] This signalled the beginning of a concerted campaign by Michael to raise the priority medical professionals gave to managing a patient's pain, something he believed many doctors neglected.

Two years after the Australian Pain Society had commissioned Paul Gross to estimate the economy-wide costs of chronic pain, he presented the preliminary report at the society's 1986 scientific meeting.[30] In *The Economic Costs of Chronic Pain in Australia,* Gross estimated the annual cost of chronic pain was $7 billion and concluded this was sufficiently large to justify federal government intervention into pain management.[53] The society shared the report with politicians and bureaucrats. Still, Michael recalls, 'No-one in political circles was listening, and some people within government ranks were openly hostile towards our attempts to put pain on the national health care agenda'.

Meanwhile, the Australian Pain Society's leaders were trying to make the society more inclusive. Some members thought it was a bit of an 'old boys' club', although this was not the view of several prominent female members. From the mid-1980s onwards nurses, psychologists, physiotherapists and dentists joined, and in 1987 Dr Jack Gerschman was the first dentist elected to the society's council. That year members elected Ms Robyn Quinn as a state councillor, paving the way for health professionals other than doctors and particularly anaesthetists, to influence the organisation.[30] As the first woman and first nurse appointed, Quinn's election marked a crucial milestone in the society's history.

In 1987, Melzack and Michael took a crucial step towards building a highly skilled pain medicine workforce by developing a curriculum for educating pain specialists. They perceived it was the right time to launch a curriculum given advances in pain medicine research and treatment, although not all IASP council members agreed with them. Michael recalls, 'It wouldn't have been possible to get consensus on a syllabus before then because we didn't know enough about pain medicine.' Several council members claimed it would be impossible to get agreement on what topics to include and which ones to exclude. Professor Howard Fields, a neurologist from the University of California San Francisco who had a bushy moustache and wore large square glasses, led a task force to create the training program.[15] Michael took part in several of its meetings. Professor Fields' skilled way of handling the often-heated exchanges and opposing views of the task force members impressed Michael.

Until then, most doctors had viewed pain as the 'poor cousin' of other medical specialties. This made it difficult to attract funding for pain services, and it deterred doctors from specialising in pain medicine. Michael believed the core curriculum enabled the profession to claim the field of pain medicine was well-defined, scientifically valid and had substance—an essential step in building forward momentum, because it gave pain medicine more credibility and prominence within the medical profession and health system.

8

PLAYING ON THE WORLD STAGE

THE pain medicine movement under John Bonica's leadership was building up a head of steam when, in 1987, Michael spent a year at Stanford University on sabbatical. The Cousins rented a house on the Stanford campus, and Michael resumed his habit of riding a bicycle to his office and the hospital. His children thought it was hilarious the way he fastened rubber bands around the bottom of his trouser legs to stop them catching in the greasy chain. But it worked, so he didn't care if it looked a bit odd. Many of Michael and Michele's friends from their three years at Stanford were still there, and they warmly welcomed them.

Michael had intended to use the year away from the day-to-day grind of his responsibilities at Flinders University to concentrate on researching the opioid hydromorphone. He planned to study the epidural administration of the analgesic in cancer pain because it had emerged as an alternative to morphine. While hydromorphone had the same potential for delayed depression of breathing as morphine, it provided pain relief quicker than morphine and cleared from the brain sooner, making it a safer option. Shortly after he arrived in Stanford, the head of Stanford University Hospital's pain clinic resigned, prompting the Dean of Medicine to ask

Michael to run the pain clinic until he appointed a replacement. Michael was disappointed because he'd been looking forward to uninterrupted research time. But he reluctantly agreed. From then on, he spent half the week overseeing the pain clinic and the rest researching hydromorphone. Still, Michael believes 'it was the best thing I've ever done. I wish I had taken a sabbatical earlier to enable me to focus more intensely on researching pain treatments without the stress of managing a university department.'

During the year at Stanford, Michael's mother Marjorie visited and flew with the Cousins to Europe for an IASP world congress in Hamburg. It was May 1987, and IASP was appointing Michael as its fifth president at the congress. Marjorie was thrilled she would be in Hamburg during her son's inauguration. The family flew from San Francisco to Zurich, then drove to Rome in the middle of a blistering heatwave. The rental car didn't have air-conditioning, so the family sweltered, but they were in high spirits, because they were heading to Rome to meet Pope John Paul II at his summer residence, Castel Gandolfo Palace.

Six years earlier, in St Peter's Square in Vatican City, a would-be assassin had shot Pope John Paul II. All four bullets had hit the pontiff. Two of them lodged in his lower intestine, just missing his vital organs, while the other two hit his left index finger and right arm. He suffered severe blood loss but remained calm. One of John Bonica's anaesthetist friends and an IASP member, Professor Corrado Manni of the Università Cattolica del Sacro Cuore in Rome, was the pontiff's anaesthetist during surgery to remove the bullets. Afterwards, the Pope suffered excruciating pain and Manni, who specialised in pain management, helped him to control it. John Bonica knew of the Pope's gratitude for the pain relief Manni had given him and being a consummate networker, even in his retirement, Bonica had written to Manni asking him whether he could organise a private audience for him with the Pope—Bonica wanted to tell the Pope about the work of IASP and the International Pain Foundation.[19]

Michele recalls the day was stifling hot and the IASP delegation of nineteen, including John and Emma Bonica, Ronald Melzack and his wife Lucy, John Liebeskind, the International Pain Foundation benefactor,

Robert Wald and his wife Toni, Professor Manni, and the Cousins family, had to wait for ages in a small room that felt like a sauna. 'Perspiration ran down our legs and we couldn't wait to return to our cars to peel off a few layers of formal clothing,' Michele said. 'But the wait was worth it. The Pope, who wore creamy white woollen robes and cut a tall slightly stooped but very fit figure, absolutely transcended us all.' Michele said the IASP delegation included people of several different religions, but Pope John Paul II eclipsed those differences and 'we all felt in awe of him'. During the audience, the Pope put his arm around Professor Manni's shoulders and said, 'This is a wonderful man; this man saved my life'.[5]

The next day, one of the Pope's staff gave Ronald Melzack a statement signed by the pontiff that addressed the work of IASP and the International Pain Foundation. In 2010, IASP's Executive Officer, Louisa Jones, said on that day in 1987, 'IASP as an organisation had come into its own'.[19]

The Cousins enjoyed six days in Hamburg. During the day while Michele, Marjorie and the children went sightseeing, Michael took part in the congress and commenced his three-year term as IASP's fifth president. Chuffed to be only the second anaesthesiologist to serve in the role—John Bonica was the first—Michael felt euphoric. But he was apprehensive about the demands of his new role, realistic that it would take a significant toll on his family.

Ronald Melzack warmly welcomed Michael to his new role at the congress and in the next edition of IASP's newsletter: 'Michael Cousins, our new president, brings many strong personal and professional qualities that will make IASP even healthier and more effective. I extend my warmest wishes to him and look forward to working with him.'[54]

This message from a colleague Michael had revered for two decades reassured him as he embarked on the challenge of leading the association through a period of rapid growth. IASP was transiting from a focus on chronic pain to one embracing acute, chronic and cancer pain and at times 'it was a bumpy ride'. In Michael's message to members in the same newsletter, he carefully laid out an ambitious agenda for his presidency. It included implementing the curriculum in pain management Howard Field had developed, increasing the research content of the journal *Pain*, strengthening IASP's relationship with the World Health Organization and contributing to the World Health Organization's global cancer pain program. He also mentioned his intention to introduce refresher courses and increase the research content of pain congresses. Reiterating his determination to increase IASP's focus on acute pain, he wrote:

<u>I would like to state quite firmly that IASP regards acute pain as being at least an equal priority to chronic pain.</u>[55]

Michael hoped that the bold underlining would make his intention to shake things up clear to the members. In an oral history interview a decade later he said, 'If people didn't like it, it was tough'.[15]

The buzz of living close to San Francisco in the 1980s energised Michael and Michele, but the suffering caused by the HIV/AIDS epidemic deeply saddened them. It was a time of intense anxiety for the city and the leading newspaper, the *San Francisco Chronicle*, frequently published articles about AIDS and the desperate need for new hospitals to cope with the scale of the crisis. 'It took the shine off living in the free atmosphere of the west coast of America for us,' Michael recalls.

During his year in Stanford, Michael combined his day job with pursuing his ambitious goals for IASP. Serving as IASP's president further reduced his leisure time, but he was happy his children played around him in the study on weekends. He became adept at multitasking, chatting with his kids about what they were doing while he worked. As soon as he took a break, he would run outside with them and play in the garden. Still, Michael regrets the way his work took him away from his children. 'I don't think I was nearly a good enough father,' he admits. 'Chris, my son, took a year off after his twins were born. I wish I had done the same.'

Michael appreciated living in the same time zone as most of his council colleagues during his sabbatical in America because speaking with them was much more manageable than trying to do it from Australia. 'It was a thrilling time to be working in pain medicine,' he recalls. 'John Bonica had created a global community of pain researchers who had previously worked on their own. Everyone shared a common purpose—we were all trying to solve the puzzle of pain. We were under John's spell. When he snapped his fingers, we jumped.'

Michael knew that once he returned to Australia, he would become frustrated with the difficulty of communicating with colleagues in the northern hemisphere. He discussed his dissatisfaction with IASP secretary, John Loeser, and the pair decided a potential solution was for Loeser to spend time in Adelaide so he and Michael could collaborate face-to-face. They wondered how to fund such an endeavour, tossing around various ideas until they landed on a workable solution—they applied for a Fulbright Scholarship to enable Loeser to spend a year on sabbatical in Adelaide.

One of IASP's council members, Mohammed Abdulmoumene, a physician who also held a position with the World Health Organization, offered to assist Michael to build a deeper relationship with the body. 'It's very complicated,' he warned. 'You have to apply. It's a lengthy process; it's very frustrating. But if you decide to do it, I think we'll make it work.' Michael jumped on his offer of help, undaunted by the obstacles ahead. 'I think we absolutely must do this. The World Health Organization has a cancer pain program, and we're now saying we should get involved in cancer pain, so we have to do it.' Kathleen Foley strongly supported the idea and so did Ronald Melzack, although some council members were less enthusiastic about it.

Navigating through WHO's dense multiple layers of bureaucracy was a slow, tortuous process. Michael had thought he could approach WHO's leaders, but he quickly learned he had to begin at the bottom and gradually work his way to the top of the organisation. Still, after three years of lobbying, Michael and his council colleagues succeeded, setting up a formal non-government organisation relationship with the World Health Organization. This alliance would lead to profound changes in global attitudes to acute and cancer pain relief and facilitate future collaborations between IASP and WHO.[15]

Throughout the 1980s, Michael's workload exploded to a level he now realises was excessive. By the mid-1980s, he had already published 139 scientific papers—equating to one every five weeks[22]—and he routinely juggled multiple research projects, took part in the federal government working group on severe pain, and wrote chapters for textbooks in his 'spare time'. Often, he found himself on call at the hospital at nights and weekends. As head of anaesthesia and intensive care, he believed it was vitally important for him to sign up for on-call duty rather than leaving it to his other colleagues.

Michael thrived on the leadership role he was playing. It exhilarated him. But as is so common with innovators and leaders, pursuing the greater good can come at the cost of sacrificing other aspects of life. He worried about the sacrifices his quest placed on his family and longed to spend more time with them all. Michael was fortunate that Michele shared his vision and backed him. She believed it was more important for her husband to focus on reducing the suffering of people with pain than 'picking up a tea towel'.[5] Michele's unwavering commitment significantly contributed to Michael's ability to pack so much into his life over so many decades. 'You just have to have the right life partner,' he said.

Meanwhile, in Australia, the National Health and Medical Research Council working group on severe pain completed its guideline and the research council published *Management of Severe Pain* in 1988. The guideline called for 'changes in training, knowledge, attitudes and practices of medical, nursing and allied professionals, along with greater public awareness of expectations in the treatment of pain'. The guideline's introduction lamented the inadequate way the Australian health system managed severe pain:

'Recent years have seen a great upsurge of interest and major advances in the management of severe pain. Tragically, many are not receiving the benefit of these advances. Severe pain is one of Australia's costliest health problems, in suffering and financial cost, affecting home and family life, work, recreation and overall quality of life for many people of all ages. Pain management in Australia can be described as "islands of enlightenment in a sea of misery".'[56]

Disappointingly, according to Michael, the guideline fell on deaf ears. 'No-one in government circles was listening despite mounting evidence of the personal, economic and societal costs of untreated pain.'

After struggling for a few years to set up and run the International Pain Foundation, Michael was forced to make a tough decision about its future. The foundation was expensive to run and hadn't attracted much funding—mainly Michael thinks because the idea involved raising money in America but spending it across the world without American control. The board members were doctors and researchers rather than fundraisers, and Michael admits he didn't have the experience he later gained in raising money from the community. When he set up the foundation, he set ambitious goals, envisioning an organisation as successful as the Red Cross.

'There was such an appalling lack of access to pain management in the world, the need was of the same magnitude as that addressed by the Red Cross.'

Sadly, the board members 'didn't have the right formula to make a success of the foundation' and Michael reluctantly shut it down in 1989.

'It was the toughest decision I've ever had to make. I didn't want to see it happen. And I think the foundation, for all of us, was a very, very challenging and I suppose, to some extent, emotional experience.'[15]

Every meeting was deeply emotional, particularly the last few. It was also painful for him because the foundation's president, John Liebeskind, was a close friend and desperately wanted to keep it running.

In 1988 the American Society of Regional Anaesthesia and Pain Medicine invited Michael to be its inaugural John J. Bonica Distinguished Lecturer. He felt deeply honoured to be the first person to present the oration. In his speech, delivered in West Virginia, Michael lamented the fact that only fifty percent of patients reported adequate pain relief following surgery. In a confident, carefully paced voice, he said, 'While surgeons usually provide pain relief in hospital for a couple of days after an operation, they rarely put in place a pain management program for their patients once they return home.' He proposed the new concept of 'acute rehabilitation'—quickly relieving pain after surgery and trauma, then continuing this care once the patient returned home.[57]

Michael suggested the benefit of an acute rehabilitation team was that it enabled patients to easily access psychologists, community nurses, physiotherapists and occupational therapists. He maintained that essential aspects of this approach were explaining an operation to a patient before the procedure to reduce their anxiety, then ensuring they got up and walked as soon as possible afterwards. He said doctors could maximise pain relief and minimise the overall dose of pain medication by administering analgesics by several routes simultaneously. For example, a patient might take one painkiller orally, an intravenous drip could deliver another drug, and an anaesthetist might inject a different medication into the epidural space.

Towards the end of the oration, Michael urged his colleagues to conduct research to identify why acute pain sometimes transitioned to chronic pain. He wanted them to discover how to prevent it happening. His speech concluded with a declaration that acute pain research offered tremendously exciting opportunities for anaesthetists, surgeons, psychologists and scientists to collaborate on ways to reduce the chance of patients developing chronic pain.

Acute pain services in Australian hospitals became common during the late 1980s, facilitated by the patient-controlled analgesia devices the Flinders team had developed. A small amount of local anaesthetic combined with a low dose of opioids provided patients with pain relief after surgery. Using epidural analgesia and these patient-controlled devices revolutionised the treatment of surgical pain. Still, it would take several years for medical staff to feel sufficiently confident about using it. Michael acknowledged the problem was 'getting the right knowledge to the right people in the right place'. A 'catch-up' problem prevailed for many years in training and educating staff. This exasperated him at the time, but he acknowledges that it always takes time for new techniques to diffuse into the hospital system.

In 1989 the *Medical Journal of Australia* invited Michael and Laurie Mather to co-author an editorial on acute pain. They titled it, 'Relief of postoperative pain: advances awaiting application', to reflect the slow pace at which medical professionals adopted new treatments.[58]

As well as focusing on pain research, Michael and a team of researchers continued his Stanford research on the toxicity of inhaled anaesthetics. At the time, drug manufacturers didn't routinely test medicines for potential toxic effects before launching them, so doctors could be using potentially dangerous drugs without realising the risks. This lack of testing gravely concerned Michael, so he assembled a team to study the toxicity of anaesthetic medications. The group included a biochemical pharmacologist, a pathologist, a surgeon and several research students. In one landmark study, they found halothane was toxic to the liver at the doses commonly used in operating theatres around the world.[59]

To Michael and John Loeser's delight, their application to the Fulbright Commission was successful, enabling Loeser to travel to Flinders University for a twelve-month sabbatical.[60] In 1989, when Loeser, his wife Karen and four-year-old son David arrived in Adelaide, Michael and Michele 'adopted' them. 'The Cousins made sure everything went smoothly for us,' Loeser said. 'They always invited us to their home for dinners and social activities with colleagues and friends.'[20] Michael turned fifty that year and Loeser was pleased he was in Australia to take part in the celebrations. During his sabbatical, Loeser spent one day each week in the Flinders pain clinic and the rest of the time researching pain medicine in the medical school library. Every Wednesday afternoon, he and Michael focused on implementing IASP's far-reaching agenda, developing guidelines for pain treatment and expanding the journal *Pain*. One possible improvement for *Pain* was publishing clinical notes, so they approached other researchers and clinicians, asking them to contribute articles to the journal. They valued their time together and fast-tracked several priority projects.[20]

A project Michael wanted to start was the development of a document on desirable characteristics of pain management centres. But several council colleagues insisted it would be impossible; it would be too sensitive and provoke too many arguments. They warned Michael of dire consequences, legal battles and people being unhappy about it. But he persisted, 'twisting John's arm' to take on this contentious project. While on sabbatical, Loeser developed a guideline, and much to his surprise when he launched it at an international pain congress, he heard no ripples of discontent.[61] Since its launch, pain centres across the globe have adopted the guideline as a standard model for interdisciplinary pain centres.[62]

While in Adelaide, Loeser and Michael collaborated on a study of different rates of spinal surgery in various regions of South Australia. The South Australian Government helped them access the patient data they needed. Loeser had previously conducted similar research in America, but he changed the design to take account of local factors. The project was a comprehensive analysis of all spinal surgery in South Australia over one year. It showed an unexplained fourfold variation in the rate of spine surgery in sixteen health care regions. The results were controversial, and the orthopaedic surgeons tried to stop Michael and Loeser from publishing them. 'The orthopods tried to push us out of shape,' but the pair persisted and eventually succeeded in sharing their results.[63] In the following years, this research contributed to reduced rates of spinal surgery in the state.

John Loeser enjoyed his time in Adelaide and appreciated the opportunity to work so closely with Michael. He believes that when Michael committed to doing something, he 'got the job done. He pulled his weight and didn't sluff it off onto anybody else'.[20]

One Christmas when Michael was IASP President, the Cousins made their annual pilgrimage by car to Palm Beach to stay with Michele's parents. The twins remember the fax machine in the second bedroom of Poppy and Trenham's compact cottage 'spewed out paper at all hours of the day and night'. The device had old thermal rolls, and thirty-metre-long faxes would emerge with IASP's logo on them. Although Michael diligently worked during the break, his children, Chris and Jane, said he still made them feel as if they were on an endless summer holiday.[64]

In early April 1990, Michael hosted the sixth world congress on pain in Adelaide. The congress marked the end of his term as IASP President. Through the congress, he aimed to attract the world's pain medicine leaders to Australia to inspire local researchers and clinicians. He also wanted to showcase the advances being made in pain medicine by Australians.

Hosting the congress in Australia worried some pain society members. They were concerned the interminable distance delegates would have to travel could act as a deterrent, making it difficult to predict the likely volume of registrations. Initially, the Adelaide psychiatrist, Issy Pilowsky, served as chair of the local arrangements committee. But he fell ill, so Dr David Cherry, director of the Flinders' pain clinic, took over the role of organising the congress. To everyone's amazement, two thousand delegates registered for the event and the pain society's membership skyrocketed during 1990.[30] Michael recalls the highlight of the congress was Ronald Melzack's presentation of the John J. Bonica Lecture, reflecting on the twenty-fifth anniversary of the revolutionary Gate Control Theory of Pain. 'This theory contributed so much to our understanding of chronic pain, enabling us to improve its treatment,' Michael said.

The participants considered the congress a magnificent success. The President's Dinner, a formal event at the end of the congress, took place in a glamorous white marquee in Highfield's garden. Ronald and Lucy Melzack, John and Emma Bonica, Patrick Wall and his wife, Vera, and many other great pioneers of pain medicine took part in the dinner. They all 'had a ball', and for years afterwards, Michael and Michele's guests would say, 'I haven't forgotten that terrific dinner at your place'. Marcia Phillips, whose husband Dr Garry Phillips was Flinders Medical Centre's head of intensive care, thought the 'house was singing', because of the floodlights shining onto its stone walls.[5]

Around the same time as the pain congress, Dr Roger Vanderfield, Royal North Shore Hospital's General Manager, approached Michael to sound him out about building an interdisciplinary pain centre at the hospital, which was going through a growth phase. A new multilevel building had recently opened, and Sydney University was keen to establish a professorial chair in anaesthesia at the hospital.

Michael had ambitious ideas about the budget he would need to establish an interdisciplinary pain centre in Sydney. By this time a tough negotiator, he demanded the hospital administrators provide him with a generous allocation of space, facilities and staff. He also had high expectations about his remuneration, refusing to settle for less. By the end of the negotiations, Vanderfield and the Northern Sydney Area Health Service chief, Dr Stuart Spring, had agreed with most of Michael's requests. Spring said Michael was one of the hardest people he had ever bargained with. 'Michael never got angry, always took the high moral ground and never let me feel the deal was sealed at any point in the discussion.' And he would often return with more demands after Spring thought he had nailed a deal. Most of the negotiations occurred over the phone or through letters rather than face-to-face. Spring recalls, 'Michael was determined to get the best deal for pain management'.[65]

9

STARTING OVER

MICHAEL started his new role as Foundation Chair of Anaesthesia and Pain Management in August 1990, commuting from Adelaide to Sydney for the first five months while his children completed the school year. When the Cousins family returned to Sydney at the end of 1990, they stayed with Poppy at her beach house at Palm Beach because Highfield was still on the market. Michele's father, Trenham, had died five years earlier and Poppy lived alone, so she enjoyed having company. Australia was in the grip of what former Labor Prime Minister, Paul Keating, called 'the recession we had to have'. The housing market was sluggish, and the stock market crash of 1987 saw share prices in Australia drop by forty percent. Unemployment and inflation were high, and massive government debt added to the nation's economic woes. 'To top it off', the State Bank of South Australia had crashed, so borrowers couldn't access funds to purchase a new house, leaving the Cousins in limbo. 'It was a tough time, but we just gritted our teeth and forged ahead,' Michael sighed.

Michele was thrilled to be back in Sydney, and she quickly reconnected with her family and friends. Michael was also pleased to be able to spend time with his mother and three siblings—Geoff, Keith and Pam Cousins.

Eventually, Highfield sold, and Michael and Michele bought a spacious home in Pymble close to their elderly mothers. The house had a garden for the children to play in, a tennis court and swimming pool. Palm Beach was a forty-minute drive away from the new house and Michael was keen to get back to weekends at the beach.

Meanwhile, in his negotiations with Roger Vanderfield and Stuart Spring, Michael had secured an agreement for Royal North Shore Hospital to partially fund a pain centre that integrated research, treatment and professional education. Sydney University didn't provide any funding, but the hospital and the Northern Sydney Area Health Service promised an annual budget of $750,000—equivalent to $1.5 million in 2020.[66]

Michael initially 'made do' with whatever space he could squeeze from the hospital's administrators. The pain clinic occupied the verandah of an old building, and two rooms that had previously been medical student quarters served as laboratories. Leaky emergency treatment rooms dating back to the 1930s housed the anaesthesia department. Despite the somewhat ramshackle accommodation, the mood at the centre was optimistic. Everyone knew they were pioneers in the nascent field of pain medicine.

Just as he'd done in Adelaide, Michael struggled with limited funding. While this was partly due to ongoing government cost-cutting, it was also because his plans for the centre were so ambitious. The area health service and hospital couldn't finance the growth targets he envisioned. Still, Stuart Spring insists the pain centre wasn't treated any differently to any other service within the health system.

'If there was a mismatch,' Spring said, 'it was Michael's ambition and the legitimate resources available given the fierce competition for health funding'.[65]

Spring recalls that Michael was better at lobbying for money than most of his colleagues and was a source of envy because the pain centre received more funding than the other departments at the hospital. Some colleagues were openly hostile towards the centre, particularly a surgeon

Michael had known since his term as an anaesthesia registrar. 'He proposed on several fronts that the idea of a pain unit be squashed,' Michael recalls. 'It was brazen that he should try to stop something that would help so many patients.'

Michele appreciated that Michael didn't bring his work stress home, even though everyone in the family could tell he felt exhausted after his gruelling days at the hospital. The twins recall that Michael, 'took things personally and worried that dealing with uncooperative bureaucrats and colleagues was taking him away from helping his patients'. Chris remembers his dad struggling through several tough patches, 'but he battled on because of his conviction that pain management was a fundamental human right. He was determined to improve pain management despite the toll it took on him'.[64]

One of Michael's first actions at Royal North Shore Hospital was to appoint his colleague from Flinders, Laurie Mather, as a professor of anaesthesia and analgesia research. As he did at Flinders, the pharmacologist played a pivotal role in getting the centre's research up and running. Once again, Mather and Michael 'started from scratch'. Their only laboratory equipment was the gas chromatograph Mather had brought with him, enabling him to measure drugs and continue the pain research he had pursued in Adelaide.[27] When John Bonica set up the pain centre in Seattle, he too had struggled with a lack of resources. But he was an astute political actor and eventually secured generous funding by developing close relationships with politicians and bureaucrats in Washington DC. Michael realised that if he was to achieve his goals he needed to redouble his efforts to build relationships with politicians on all sides of the political spectrum.

To raise enough funds to construct a purpose-designed pain management centre, Michael formed an appeal board that included prominent community members. The businessman Rick Turner led the group. During its first fundraising stage, the appeal board raised $1.3 million, including a generous donation from the health insurance company, Medical Benefits Fund Australia (MBF). Thanks to this vigorous fundraising, Royal North Shore Hospital officially launched stage one of the Centre for Anaesthesia and Pain Management Research on 14 May 1991.[67]

Michael modelled the new centre on what he had witnessed at the University of Washington and applied his learnings from running the Flinders Medical Centre's pain centre. He was energised, but also depleted by the sheer number of tasks on his to-do list each day. Still, he doggedly pursued his agenda, intent on building a world-class facility.

Meanwhile, Jonathan, Chris and Jane were growing up, and life at home was hectic. Michele acted as the primary disciplinarian because she spent so much time with the children, and Michael served as the family's peacemaker. Jane recalls that when a dispute arose, her father would patiently listen to everyone's point of view, then find a fair solution. 'Mum and Dad were big believers in not going to bed angry or upset with somebody,' Jane said. 'Dad urged us to resolve our differences well before bedtime.'[68]

Chris describes his father as a 'warm, loving, calming force' in the household, firm rather than strict. 'Dad taught us values such as being honest, kind and looking after people.'[64] The boys also learned 'olde-worlde manners' from their father, such as pulling out the dining chair and opening car doors for women. If Michael's children had a problem they couldn't work out, he would sit with them, draw up a pros and cons list, and try to solve the problem logically. 'Don't sweat the small stuff,' was a favourite piece of advice, and whenever his children worked on a project, he told them to 'Remember the Five Ps,' the formula for success his father, Hedley, had taught him.

On weekends, Michael urged his children to get up and play outside the way he had done as a child. He had freely roamed through the bush at Killara and spent hours rocketing down the steep hill of his street on a homemade billy cart. One of his favourite sayings was: 'Get up. Get outside. Get some fresh air'. He was a big believer in exercise and fresh air, considering both to be 'good for the soul', and this belief was among several that drove his quest to improve pain management. He wanted everyone to be able to enjoy the benefits of being active.[68]

One of the patients whom Michael helped to remain active despite her crippling pain was Pamela Nock, who struggled with chronic neck, shoulder and back pain. She suffered from haemochromatosis, a hereditary condition that causes the body to absorb too much iron from the diet. The tissues and organs store the excess iron, damaging the joints and causing arthritis. The condition can also trigger migraines, and Pamela's were so severe her GP regularly visited her at home to inject a drug to stop the vomiting and pain. Michael explained to Pamela that there was no cure for her chronic pain, but he promised her he could give her temporary relief and reduce the impact chronic pain had on her life.

Every three weeks Michael injected the anti-inflammatory drug cortisone into Pamela's most painful joints. These injections gave her relief, but sometimes within a week, the familiar pain returned in full force. Another technique Michael tried was radio-frequency lesioning, which involved using small needles carrying electrical energy to heat a nerve to eighty degrees Celsius. After two to three minutes, the nerve would stop carrying pain signals for up to the eighteen months it took to regrow.[69]

Pamela valued the way Michael always encouraged her to persevere, no matter how much the pain affected her. When it stopped her from playing tennis or working on her family's farm, he suggested she take up painting and ceramics. Pamela says these new hobbies took away the strain of not being able to play sport and do the things she most enjoyed.

Pamela liked the friendly atmosphere at the clinic, and she appreciated the way Michael and the nursing team were always willing to 'go the extra mile to help the patients'. She said that in reducing her pain, Michael made her life seem a little easier. 'I appreciated his kindness, empathy and compassion, and he offered me hope; he helped me to see the light at the end of the tunnel.'

After every procedure, Pamela valued Michael's habit of checking on her multiple times before allowing her to go home. 'Michael was busy running in and out of the operating theatre and looking after several patients simultaneously, so I was grateful he was so caring towards me.' Pamela felt Michael truly listened to her and often spoke with her on the phone after hours if she needed his advice.

'The name Michael Cousins will always be at the top of the chart for anything to do with pain,' she said.[70]

The growing demand for pain management services and the centre's rapidly expanding research program quickly raised the need for more staff and space. Michael recalls the centre was understaffed and team members felt 'continually beleaguered', as though they 'worked on a half-empty tank—sometimes even an empty tank'. As funding improved, Michael prioritised the recruitment of highly qualified scientists and clinicians. As he had done at Flinders University, he searched the globe for researchers with a keen interest in clinical practice and teaching. He collaborated with Sydney University colleagues, recruiting critical members of the anatomy and pharmacology departments. He was delighted when prominent neuroscientist, Professor Arthur Duggan, formerly of the University of Edinburgh, joined the centre. He was equally pleased when Dr Richard Bandler, a professor of anatomy and pain research, and Dr Kevin Keay, a senior lecturer in anatomy and pain research, also accepted his job offers.

Dr Allan Molloy, who joined the centre as a pain medicine specialist in 1992, said the clinic had a convivial manner despite its rudimentary accommodation. 'All the staff were immensely caring towards the patients,' he recalls, 'and I appreciated how Michael had set up a weekly meeting for staff to talk about the latest research discoveries and journal articles'. Molloy also enjoyed the meetings team members had after assessing each patient. 'We all met to tailor a treatment plan for every patient in true interdisciplinary style.'[71]

One of the medical students at the hospital was Dr Marc Russo, who is now a specialist pain medicine physician and spinal stimulation researcher. Russo recalls that Michael was kind and compassionate with his patients and came across to the medical students as 'old school'. 'That old school professor who was extremely knowledgeable, extremely in command and confident,' Russo said. 'I remember his gentleness with the patients, and that's not something I saw necessarily every day, especially from many of the other professors who usually had a retinue of registrars, residents, interns and nurses trailing behind.' Russo claims being on a ward round with some professors was like being at the theatre—'a bit of show, barking commands or whatever to the junior staff, and it would be quite a hurried affair. But Michael wasn't like that. During ward rounds he exuded calmness and confidence and spent time with his patients.'[72]

When the twins were eleven, Michael won a grant to travel overseas for three weeks giving lectures about pain medicine. He and Michele thought this would be an ideal opportunity to combine work with a visit to Canada to see their oldest son, James, who was working in the ski fields at Lake Louise. They flew to Seattle and stayed with John Loeser and his family. Then they hired a Lincoln Town car and Michael drove through heavy snow in the dark to Revelstoke, high in the mountains. Their hotel had a hot tub, so after warming up in the steaming water the Cousins, including Michael in his black Speedos, jumped outside into the snow. The next day they drove to Lake Louise. Once they'd left James, they travelled to Calgary. While Michael gave lectures and met with his pain colleagues there, Michele and the children went sightseeing and to the zoo. Canada was bitterly cold and wet, so they were relieved the destinations of Michael's next presentations were hotter—Trinidad and Barbados, then Miami.

After Michael returned to Australia, he and Mather became so exasperated with the pain centre's funding shortfall they threatened to resign. And they meant it. Fortunately, this prompted hospital administrators to 'loosen the purse strings', and some more funding flowed. But it was never enough to meet the increasing patient demand for services and Michael's aggressive growth plans.

During the early 1990s, the stomach cramps Michael had experienced since childhood often troubled him and he felt unwell. One day Michele shared her concerns about his health with her bridge partner who suggested the problem could be food intolerance and that the allergy unit at Sydney's Royal Prince Alfred Hospital might be able to help. Michael made an appointment to see Professor Rob Loblay and the head dietitian, Dr Anne Swain, who recommended he start an elimination diet. For the first couple of weeks, all he ate was iceberg lettuce, boiled potatoes, white rice and peeled pears.

Michael kept a diary during the prescribed three-month diet and once it finished Swain told him he had reacted to salicylates and amines. From then on, the family ate 'strange things' like chokos that the twins called 'chuckos'. Beer and wine contain salicylate, so Michael switched to drinking whisky. Over the years he became an aficionado, preferring single malts such as Laphroaig and Highland Park. The contents of Michael's lunch box would become a running joke at the pain centre. After his diagnosis, Michele packed a lunch of rice cakes with cashew butter, a simple salad, boiled eggs and a can of four bean mix for him. Michael would try to crunch his rice cakes quietly during lunch meetings to prevent disturbing the presenter, but it was an uphill battle because they were so crispy.

To this day, Michael firmly believes some of the most significant advances in modern medicine—such as the development of penicillin and the invention of the cochlear ear implant—resulted from a genuine interaction between clinicians and scientists. But one huge challenge he faced was convincing the scientists who studied cells and the neurophysiology of pain to collaborate with the clinicians who treated patients. And vice versa. This critical issue also concerned John Bonica, who had tried to address it by establishing IASP as an interdisciplinary organisation.

Over the years, Bonica and Michael often discussed this problem. Both knew that solving it was central to the advancement of pain medicine.

10

ADVANCING PAIN RESEARCH

THE integration of basic and clinical research attracted many talented researchers and clinicians to Royal North Shore Hospital's pain centre. The basic pain research program focused on the mechanisms associated with injury to major nerves or the spinal cord. The clinical research program focused on three major areas: pain after surgery and trauma, cancer pain and chronic pain. While the cancer pain research investigated ways of treating severe pain associated with the disease, the chronic pain research initially concentrated on spinal cord injuries and the outcome of various pain management approaches.

In 1992, keen to combine research with clinical care, Dr Philip Siddall joined the pain centre at Royal North Shore Hospital. During his interview for the job, Siddall mentioned his interest in researching nerve pain. Michael asked him whether he would like to start a research program on spinal cord injury pain, the head of the hospital's spinal unit having previously asked Michael if he could study the condition because his patients suffered so much pain. The idea excited Siddall; it was a brand-new area of medicine. 'No-one had done much research on spinal cord injury pain anywhere across the globe.'[73]

As soon as he arrived at the hospital, Siddall started his spinal cord injury research program. One day while chatting with another of the researchers at the pain centre, Dr David Taylor, they discussed the need for consensus about the classification of the various types of pain that occurred after a spinal cord injury. This lack of agreement caused confusing variations in how medical professionals recorded the condition, making it difficult to assess the magnitude of the problem. It also hampered studies of different treatment approaches.

Siddall, Taylor and Michael believed that both research and treatment would benefit from a consistent classification system, one that accurately identified various pain forms, so they set to work creating one. They divided spinal cord injury pain into musculoskeletal, internal organ, nerve and other types of pain, then further subdivided nerve pain into two categories. After completing the classification, they published an article describing their approach in the influential journal, *Spinal Cord*.[74] The international response surprised and delighted them. The classification system seemed to resonate with clinicians and researchers worldwide and, because it brought consensus to the terminology used in describing pain after spinal cord injury, it soon became the most widely used classification system in the pain medicine and spinal cord injury communities.[73]

Encouraged by the rapturous initial response to their classification system, Siddall, Michael and their team of researchers continued with studies on pain after spinal cord injury. They developed a new rat model of nerve pain,[75] and in one investigation, showed that genetic changes occurred in cells above the level of the spinal cord injury.[76] In patients, the team tested whether opioids and non-opioid drugs delivered via the intrathecal space—the fluid-filled area between the innermost layer covering the spinal cord and the middle layer—relieved spinal cord injury nerve pain and found that if they combined morphine with the blood pressure reducing medication clonidine, the heightened pain sensitivity was eased.[77] From then on, they implanted tiny pumps into some of their patients, enabling the delivery of a continuous dose of morphine and clonidine into the spinal fluid.

In another study, the team found 150 to 600 mg each day of the anticonvulsant drug pregabalin relieved spinal cord injury nerve pain.[78] It also improved sleep, anxiety and patient wellbeing. Michael was tremendously excited by this research. Up until the mid-1990s he had felt frustrated by the poor response to his attempts to treat severe nerve pain in patients with a spinal cord injury, but now they were on the cusp of a new era.

Significantly, the team also pursued spinal cord injury pain in the clinic, following up patients from the emergency department through the rehabilitation phase to five years after injury. In this study, the researchers found eighty-one percent of the patients reported pain.[79] Musculoskeletal pain was the most common type, with nearly sixty percent of patients describing their pain as severe or excruciating. Those with pain in internal organs, such as the heart, lungs, pancreas or intestines, were most likely to rate their pain as severe or excruciating.

In mid-1993, Michael's brother, Keith, suddenly died of a heart attack. He was sixty-eight. Michael was engulfed by grief. He was proud of Keith. Like Hedley and Geoff Cousins, Keith was one of Australia's advertising titans. He had retired as chair of Australia's largest advertising agency, George Patterson, in 1984. One advertising industry chief, Terry Connaghan, said: 'Keith Cousins was a friend, counsellor and powerbroker to leading politicians of all persuasions, to the leading companies, and a very long list of businessmen. He used his position at George Patterson to further the cause of the advertising industry and was unselfish in the amount of time he gave to that cause.'[80] This trait seemed to run in the Cousins' family.

The following year, while Michael struggled to come to terms with Keith's death, two momentous events occurred. In recognition of his contributions to pain medicine and anaesthesia, Michael received a Member of the Order of Australia award (AM) from the nation's Governor-General. He was proud to receive the honour but believed it belonged to the entire pain centre team.

The other momentous event occurred when Michael's phone rang early one morning in August 1994. It was John Bonica.

'I'm dying, son,' the older man announced, his voice soft and shaky.

From the day they had met in 1973, Michael and Bonica had worked well together, frequently telephoning and faxing and seeing each other at IASP council meetings and congresses. Bonica had always encouraged Michael when the younger doctor's energy was flagging from his constant battles. The older professor generously shared tips based on his own experiences and boosted Michael's confidence when he was faced with what seemed like 'insurmountable obstacles'.

Michael offered to jump onto the next flight to America to say goodbye to Bonica in person.

'It's too late,' Bonica whispered. 'I will die tomorrow. Michael, my friend, it's been good knowing you.'

Michael was inconsolable. He deeply valued his friendship with his long-time mentor and to lose him so soon after Keith's sudden loss left an enormous hole in his heart. Both deaths would weigh on him for many years, as had Hedley's passing and that of his precious son, Richard, a decade earlier.

Nonetheless, Michael was happy that John Bonica had the satisfaction of seeing the specialty of pain medicine come of age. 'Few people in medicine these days are the father of a brand-new field. John Bonica was one of them, and I owe so much to him.'

11

CHRONIC PAIN: MICHAEL'S PATIENTS SHARE THEIR STORIES

ONE of the pain centre's primary research and treatment focus areas has been and continues to be chronic pain. Pain professionals take several treatment approaches to manage chronic pain, depending on each patient's circumstances. Neuroplasticity research has revealed the brain and nervous system are constantly changing, and the brain can learn to turn down the volume of pain signals.[81] Hence, various treatments aim to help the nervous system return to normal pain processing so the person living with pain can improve their day-to-day functioning and quality of life.

One of Michael's earliest patients at the pain clinic was a woman named Robyn M. She had suffered decades of neck pain and headaches following a car accident. Over the years, she had endured several neck operations, and her GP kept prescribing progressively higher doses of pain medication. But 'nothing helped', and the drugs made her feel drowsy. After seeing her children off to school each morning, she spent the rest of the day lying on her bed with ice packs placed along one side of her neck to reduce the crippling pain. She 'limped from one commitment to the next, always accompanied by the familiar pain'.[82]

Robyn appreciated how Michael explained the nature of chronic pain and admitted his inability to cure it. But he assured her he would do everything in his power to relieve it and reduce its impact on her life. He suggested he implant a morphine pump into her spine to deliver a continuous but tiny dose of morphine.

'The morphine pump worked and was my salvation,' Robyn said. 'It saved my sanity and was a lifesaver.'[82]

Every five weeks Robyn returns to the clinic for a top-up, and over the last twenty-six years, the pump has enabled her to live a relatively 'normal' life. Before this treatment, Robyn felt her 'life slipping away, and it seemed like one terrible agonising day after another'. But 'those days are over' much to her relief. 'It's miraculous! Absolutely miraculous!' she says. 'Meeting Michael Cousins changed my life.'[82]

Although complications sometimes occurred and it hasn't been all smooth sailing, Robyn is now much better and lives a good life. The morphine dose, which was minuscule when Michael implanted the pump, has increased over the years because her body has adapted to the medication. But Robyn has experienced no other side effects.

Michael also implanted a morphine pump to help Jaswir Grewal manage his lower back pain. Jaswir had a twenty-year history of back pain caused by decades of working as a banana grower and motor mechanic. Pain ruled his life and 'took over everything'.[83] He had endured three spinal fusion operations in the 1980s, but they didn't relieve his pain, so in 1992 his GP referred him to the clinic. Michael, Allan Molloy and the interdisciplinary team assessed Jaswir. Their advice surprised him. Michael suggested he implant a morphine pump into Jaswir's spine. Jaswir agreed to this surgery, excited that it might be a 'light at the end of the tunnel'.[83] Once the pump was in place, it provided him with pain relief for ten years.

However, for Jaswir, the morphine triggered unpleasant side effects. His pupils dilated at night, so if he tried to drive his car at dusk or when it was dark, he couldn't tell which lane oncoming cars were in. So he stopped driving at night. He also experienced mood swings, and his irritability seriously upset his wife. Over time, his body adapted to the morphine and he required progressively higher doses. Still, the pump reduced his pain and enabled him to live a better life, so he accepted its downsides. But then disaster struck. The pump migrated and was about to rupture the surface of his skin, forcing Michael to remove it.

Life was tough for Jaswir without the morphine pump. Michael suggested he take part in an interdisciplinary pain management program the pain centre's psychologist, Dr Michael Nicholas, had pioneered. Nicholas had joined the centre in 1994 when it still occupied the dilapidated verandah. He had previously developed a four-week inpatient program for people with chronic pain at St Thomas' Hospital in London, and once Royal North Shore Hospital's pain clinic moved to 'Level Nine' of the new tall brown building, he introduced a three-week outpatient version of the program.[84]

Nicholas recruited the physiotherapist Lois Tonkin, nurse Lee Beeston and clinical psychologist Tim Sharp to run the program. Allan Molloy provided initial medical care for the participants. At the beginning, the team scurried around searching for patients funded by workers' compensation companies to ensure the pain clinic could afford to pay its staff.[85] Early on the team realised they couldn't rely on government funding, so Michael and Nicholas made multiple visits to workers compensation companies and NSW WorkCover seeking their financial support. The insurers were keen to get injured employees back to work to reduce compensation payouts, so they provided funding for some patients to attend the program.

Michael also approached foundations and philanthropists, many of whom provided generous support. This funding enabled the program to grow, and Nicholas built up the team to include several physiotherapists, clinical psychologists and nurses. The team members took an interdisciplinary approach, jointly designing a treatment plan for each participant and regularly updating each other on the participants' progress and their management plan.

This program, which Nicholas named ADAPT (Active Day-Patient Treatment), was based on a cognitive-behavioural treatment approach to chronic pain and included education about the underlying mechanisms contributing to pain, carefully graded exercises and training in pain self-management strategies such as pacing, flare-up management and relaxation. It aimed to maximise participants' ability to live well with chronic pain by equipping them with tools to minimise the impact of the pain on their lives.

ADAPT set out to help people get from 'where they were when they started the program to where they wanted to be' by gradually increasing their function without aggravating the pain. Participants worked towards achieving their own goals to help them get their life back on track. 'That requires a person to achieve and maintain a healthy lifestyle despite pain,' Nicholas explains, 'which often means dealing with depression, anxiety and the effects of prolonged stress. It also includes improving sleep quality, physical functioning and fitness.'[84]

The ADAPT team encouraged participants to reduce and eventually stop taking unhelpful pain medications and, at the same time, increase their activity level, which risked aggravating the pain. The way to prevent a flare up of pain is to 'pace'—gradually build up exercise or an activity so the body can adjust to it. According to data from the ADAPT program, if people pace well, they not only reduce their disability, but they have less pain.[84]

Jaswir Grewel found ADAPT's team members welcoming, but he struggled at first when they tried to teach him to meditate. He found it difficult to stop thinking about the pain when he was in a room with fifteen other patients, many of whom 'jiggled around, groaned and sighed' because of their pain. But he 'hung in there' and found it helpful. The exercises initially caused his pain to flare up, so the physiotherapist adapted them for him. Jaswir enjoyed learning about nutrition, how to cope with pain and how to walk and lift correctly. It helped him to 'live a better life'.[83]

Michael also suggested to his patient, Pamela Nock, that she take part in ADAPT. He thought the program would help her manage the arthritic pain and migraines that resulted from her hemochromatosis. The lectures about pain and its management helped Pamela to stop feeling nervous and worried about her pain. She also learned to meditate, and the physiotherapist encouraged her to increase her physical activity, something she had avoided because of her pain. 'ADAPT helped me to live a normal life,' she said.[70]

Symantha Liu first met Michael in the mid-1990s having suffered from chronic neck pain and migraines since she was five years old. Michael offered Symantha several treatment options, including nerve blocks and cutting-edge medications. Some treatments worked better than others or lasted longer than others, but she felt hopeful. Michael treated her with dignity, giving her the courage to keep trying. Over decades of seeking help, Symantha had felt frustrated; she rarely met doctors who showed genuine compassion, or who had an authentic understanding of the heavy burden persistent pain sufferers lived with every day. She was overwhelmed by Michael's kind and caring manner and his ability to really 'listen' to his patients. She said he changed her life.[86]

Symantha later enrolled in ADAPT. She found its communal nature immensely helpful and appreciated the support of other participants. They gave her the confidence to keep going during the more confronting moments of the program. ADAPT 'wasn't easy'; it challenged Symantha to think about her lifestyle and coping mechanisms in entirely different ways. For several years, doctors had told her to ignore the pain whenever she found herself in an uncontrollable situation, such as on an aeroplane. They said she would panic less if she tricked her mind and pretended the pain was not there or was not as severe as she thought it to be. But this advice had significant limitations. Once she reached her threshold, no amount of 'ignoring' would take away the overwhelming rush of crippling pain.[86]

ADAPT's approach taught Symantha a new coping strategy called desensitisation—the polar opposite of the 'ignoring pain strategy' she had traditionally used. Desensitisation involves learning not to react to pain in a negative way. This retrains the way the brain thinks about pain, which can improve the experience of pain and pain levels.[69] ADAPT's psychologist urged Symantha to lean into her pain and embrace it, no matter how severe it felt on a scale from one to ten. This took courage, immense will and 'much, much practice', but Symantha valued the support of the pain centre staff. Their encouragement was paramount in the early stage of 'unlearning' and breaking the old habits she had relied on for decades. She noticed a strong pull back to her familiar coping mechanisms, things she knew would help even if only five times out of ten. She found desensitising confronting, especially when first trying to master it. It took her a long time, and today she still at times experiences moments of struggle or extreme anxiety. But she believes that 'pushing through and embracing the pain in some strange way is a better method for coping'. It gives her more self-control.[86]

Charm Frend, who was born with a degenerative disc disease and had endured ten back operations, also found ADAPT immensely beneficial. On the day of her initial assessment, Charm was impressed with how the pain centre's team developed an integrated plan of action for her. For years, she had been trying to get her specialists to talk to her GP, physio and care group team, but to no avail. She appreciated how Michael, the physio and psychologist discussed her condition as a team and developed a management plan based on her individual needs.[87]

On her first day of the ADAPT program, Charm didn't feel ready to have people tell her the pain wouldn't go away and she had to learn to function despite the pain. The initial week was challenging. Charm wasn't sure about it, especially trying to accept that chronic pain couldn't be cured. However, she was surprised when other participants shared their stories; until then she hadn't realised her experiences were so commonplace. It showed her she wasn't alone. After hearing everyone's stories, Charm realised they were all the same, even though they each had unique problems in dealing with chronic pain.

During the first day of ADAPT, the physiotherapist videotaped the participants walking down a hospital corridor. She repeated this procedure at the end of the program. Charm's progress astonished her because she hadn't expected to improve so much. 'On the first day, all the participants walked with bent necks, hunched shoulders and slumped backs, and they looked depressed and tired,' Charm said. 'But by the end of the three weeks, they were all standing tall and looked much better.'[87]

After finishing the program, Charm felt more confident about her day-to-day functioning. ADAPT helped her understand why her body was doing what it was doing. It didn't make her want to run out and apply for a full-time job, but it did help her realise if she paced her activities, she was able to do a little more than previously. She felt more assured of coping well from one day to the next. She no longer felt like 'wallowing at home all day' as she had in the past. It also gave her the courage to talk about her condition. Charm had always felt guilty when she woke in the morning with severe back pain and cancelled her swimming coaching client, but after ADAPT, she told her clients about her pain and why she needed to scrap their lesson.

Charm maintains she is more socially active now and less withdrawn. ADAPT gave her the confidence to admit to her friends when she was having an awful day and preferred to remain at home. While Charm feels ADAPT made her more positive, she realises she still experiences slumps, 'but that's a bit of who I am'. After doing the program, she stopped grieving for the things the pain prevented her from doing. 'Michael and the team gave me the certainty I could cope with my pain. I'm not as crippled as I thought I was. I thought I was useless. I now have the assurance that I can put myself out there a bit. I can be of use to someone.'[87]

My own experience with chronic pain introduced me to Michael in 2005. I came to ADAPT after a fifteen-year history of debilitating daily migraines that had started a decade after some young men pushed me off my bicycle from their speeding car. The force of impact was so strong it propelled me into the air, and I landed on my head before rolling headfirst down the road. I was knocked unconscious and woke up in hospital with excruciating neck pain. Fortunately, I soon recovered and within a few months returned to cycling, tennis, sailing and bushwalking.

Unfortunately, my pain-free state was short-lived. In the early 1990s, I regularly flew from Sydney to other capital cities in Australia as part of my job. I was studying business at night and spent the idle hours on planes reading my textbooks. About half an hour into each flight, a pain like an electric shock would shoot up the back of my neck and head. The pain eventually spread upwards, fanning out until it covered the entire back of my head and temples. Within a few months, the pain I experienced in planes became more regular. It was most severe after playing my piano and cello or going sailing. My physiotherapist put it down to early onset arthritis caused by flying off my bike at high speed all those years ago.

Meanwhile, I started a job in Canberra as a ministerial adviser. Each morning, I would feel shooting pains running up the back of my head, accompanied by waves of intense nausea. My eyes felt gritty, as if they were full of sand, and I yearned for them to explode to release the mounting pressure inside them. Usually, before the pain started, I noticed squiggly lines, blotches and blurry patches in front of my eyes. Often when the pain was at its worst, I couldn't think of the words I wanted to say. My mouth also refused to form the right words, as if the messages weren't getting through from my brain to the muscles in my face. It infuriated my boss and some colleagues.

After returning to Sydney, I despaired of ever being free of pain and nausea. I had forgotten what being pain-free felt like and was elated on the rare days I had a break. I consulted an endless round of medical specialists and health professionals, but none of them helped much. Eventually, I stopped doing all the things I loved because they triggered migraines.

While on the endless merry-go-round of visits to doctors, I finally ended up at Royal North Shore Hospital's pain clinic. I sat in the waiting room feeling hopeful but also nervous. I had tried so many treatments, and none had worked. After a while, a man with neatly combed grey hair who looked like he was in his mid-sixties appeared in the brightly lit corridor. He wore a dark navy suit, pristine white shirt and navy tie with red diagonal stripes. His black leather shoes were glossed to a high shine and when he smiled, I noticed he had braces on his teeth.

'Hi, I'm Professor Michael Cousins. Sorry, I'm running so late. Clinic days are always crazily busy. Please follow me.'

We walked through the clinic with its wide corridors, freshly painted walls and bright lights. Michael led me into his office, pulling out an upholstered chair and inviting me to sit down. He sat in a black leather office chair, cupped his hands and knitted his eyebrows. 'I've read your notes, and it sounds like you've been having a tough time.' We talked for an hour. Afterwards, in a soft but confident voice, Michael explained what was happening in my central nervous system and why I lived a life of almost constant pain. As our conversation ended, he looked me directly in the eyes and smiled. 'I'm confident we can help you. It'll take time and be a long journey, but we'll do it together.'

Every couple of months after that initial consultation I saw Michael at the pain clinic. He trialled a range of medications to determine whether they would help prevent my migraines. It was a process of trial and error, and with each medication I brimmed with hope, only to have it dashed when it failed to stop the migraines or triggered nasty side effects. But Michael never gave up on me. He stayed the course despite my disappointing response to his repeated attempts to relieve my pain.

Two months after Michael suggested I participate in ADAPT, I arrived at the pain clinic for the first day of the three-week program. I stepped inside the seminar room, then abruptly stopped. Ahead loomed exercise bikes, a treadmill, small hand weights, a set of steps and a mountain of blue yoga mats. I quivered, the knot in my stomach tightening. A whiteboard that someone had tried to clean but still retained faded writing and diagrams filled the space at the front of the room. I edged towards one of the blue plastic chairs, arranged in a semicircle that took up most of the free space. Several men and women perched on the chairs. Most of them fidgeted or jiggled around, and their shoulders sagged. Their faces were pallid, and dark circles hung under their eyes.

One of the participants said hello and asked me my name. Two others stopped their conversation and greeted me.

'What brings you here,' a burly man covered in tattoos said. 'I have a crook back.'

'Chronic migraine,' I stammered.

'Me too,' said a woman with soft grey curls. She wore black tailored slacks and a pink cardigan.

I heard stories of decades-long battles with crippling back pain and getting by on a cocktail of opioid medications that left my companions living what one young man described as 'a blurry half-life'. Despite the opioids, they still suffered unimaginable pain, and were unable to work, sleep, play with their children or resume other pre-injury activities. They grieved for what they had lost.

At nine o'clock, two staff arrived and introduced themselves. One was a psychologist and the other a physiotherapist. They described the ADAPT program and its structure. Then the psychologist talked about chronic pain—what it was, what caused it and how it differed from acute pain. He said acute pain and chronic pain require different treatment approaches because of their differing underlying causes.

Then he dropped his voice. 'Chronic pain doesn't have a cure, but we'll teach you how to manage your pain and reduce its impact on your life.'

Some participants shuffled in their seats and sighed; others looked crestfallen. The psychologist said one of ADAPT's aims was to help patients taper off their pain medications. At that point, the room erupted. I heard a collective gasp as if the walls had taken a deep breath, then shuddered. A few participants heckled the psychologist. One patient stormed out, slamming the door behind him. Another paced around his chair. Despite the hostile atmosphere, the psychologist stood his ground and continued his presentation. He said he would teach us cognitive behavioural therapy techniques that would help us change how we thought about and dealt with pain, enabling us to live a good life despite it.

After the psychologist's talk, the physio said it was time for an exercise session. She handed out sheets of paper with a list of exercises printed down one side and a grid on the other side and explained that we would have two exercise sessions at the clinic each day and one at home. We were to record how many repetitions we did of each exercise and its intensity. Gradually we would increase the number of repetitions and intensity by a tiny amount. In this way, we'd build up our strength and our body's tolerance to the exercise. We started by gently stretching individual muscle groups then progressed to strengthening exercises using the hand weights. The exercise session continued for about forty minutes and included aerobic exercises such as pedalling the exercise bike, trotting on the treadmill and climbing stairs. I enjoyed it. Surprisingly, it didn't hurt my neck or trigger a migraine. Finally, I felt I was making progress.

ADAPT taught me to stop catastrophising and to believe I had the power to change how I reacted to pain. It was life-changing. While migraines remain my constant companion, they are now less debilitating and far less frequent. The way I deal with them is also different. When I spark a flare-up by writing for too long or swimming too far, I use the skills I learned in ADAPT, such as pacing, to turn down the volume of pain signals racing through my malfunctioning nervous system. For years I have practised the exercises every day, adding gentle Qigong and yoga routines to keep it fresh. I also use desensitisation, which has become central to my daily routine.

The model of care Michael advocated through ADAPT and the pain clinic's interdisciplinary approach was a revelation to many GPs and pain specialists in Australia—even in the 2000s. Some pain physicians first learned of interdisciplinary pain management when they visited Royal North Shore Hospital's pain clinic years into their career. Fortunately for the pain medicine physician, Marc Russo, he was able to visit it during his specialist training.

When Russo returned to Royal North Shore Hospital – he had been a medical student there – he caught the lift to the pain clinic, on level nine of the hospital's old brown building. The first things he noticed when he stepped into the pain clinic's treatment room were the pale lemon curtains, crisp white sheets on the modern hospital beds, and the positive vibe. Patients and staff chatted and some quietly laughed. It astonished him because in the 1980s and early 1990s when he had worked in pain clinics in Australia and overseas, they were antiquated or dilapidated—Nissen huts left over from the Vietnam war and an original Victorian poorhouse converted to medical use. In one hospital, the receptionist on the ground floor gave patients directions to the pain clinic: 'When you reach the basement turn left,' she said, 'otherwise you'll end up in the morgue.'

Russo recalls some pain clinics were a sad place where the people whom no-one else could help ended up. 'They were the patients that either medicine couldn't help, or often, unfortunately, the ones whom medicine had harmed. I remember on occasions processions of people in wheelchairs on ridiculous doses of opioids enduring the most miserable lives.'[72]

Russo said he was lucky. 'I was taught pain medicine in the era when Michael and other colleagues around Australia had transformed assessment and care into an interdisciplinary model.' Russo noted that many of his mentors – early pioneers like Michael – had done it tough seeing patients by themselves with little to no help from physios, psychologists and nurses. Some of them had only been able to work in the pain clinic by sacrificing their non-clinical admin day and converting it into a pain clinic consulting day or if they were a visiting medical officer they offered their services pro bono. 'We had to beg, borrow or steal support from physios and psychologists who were busy providing services throughout the main hospital,' he added.[72]

'What Michael brought was interdisciplinary care where a patient was seen simultaneously by a pain specialist, a physio, a social worker and a psychologist,' Russo explains. 'After each team member had assessed the patient, they got together to discuss the treatment plan, then the pain specialist debriefed the patient.'[72]

Russo said Michael held up interdisciplinary pain management as the benchmark, and other pain clinics throughout Australia gradually adopted it. 'Michael rewrote the minimum basic standard for pain management. It solidified the role for allied health professionals inside a pain clinic. You can question whether it is the most cost-effective model and is it the most time-efficient model, but there are several ways you can slice and dice the health care dollar. Before Michael introduced interdisciplinary pain management in Australia, we had only tokenistic representation of allied health care. I think it's fair to say he virtually single handedly changed that in this country.' Russo paused. 'I'm not suggesting that Michael invented this from scratch. He himself was exposed to it through John Bonica, so it is an extension of Bonica's pioneering work. Each generation builds on the experience of the previous generation and Michael embraced what Bonica taught him and introduced it in Australia.'[72]

Sadly, not all people with chronic pain benefit from interdisciplinary pain management programs. Allan Molloy maintains it can be difficult for a person with chronic pain who has been off work and on workers' compensation for an extended period to change from being a passive recipient of health services to one who self-manages their pain. This reaction is especially true if they have tried multiple approaches that have all failed to relieve their pain. 'To transform them into using self-management, into someone who's enjoying their life, can be a challenge,' he said. Molloy admits that participants may be fearful the exercises will cause their pain to flare up, and sometimes they are sceptical, even cynical of the program's cognitive behavioural therapy.[71]

Still, over the years, thousands of people have benefited from interdisciplinary pain management and Michael fervently believes in its value.

'Interdisciplinary pain management is the gold standard of care for chronic pain,' he insists.

12

THE TROUBLING TRANSITION

AS well as studying chronic pain, Michael continued to investigate acute pain and its treatment. 'Poorly managed acute pain can transition to chronic pain, so our team was eager to develop better treatments for acute pain to prevent this from happening,' he explains. One of Michael's mentors, Professor Tom Reeve, was a councillor of Australia's National Health and Medical Research Council. Reeve's colleagues admired the way he continually searched for opportunities to improve the human condition. Michael often spoke with Reeve about the need for the Australian government to take a greater interest in pain management. Reeve petitioned the research council, urging it to appoint Michael as a councillor. 'Much to my delight, they did it,' Michael said.

Reeve suggested the research council establish a working party to examine the scientific literature on managing acute pain. The council agreed, appointing Michael as chair. 'I got going straightaway,' he recalls. 'I knew it would fill my nights and weekends for many years, but it was an urgent priority, and I felt compelled to do it.'

Michael's first step was to invite leading pain management professionals from around Australia to participate in multidisciplinary committees. He asked the committee members to study the scientific evidence in their area of responsibility. By this time, pain research had taken off and researchers were feverishly publishing their latest findings. Every night, Michael carried big bundles of research papers home from the hospital. 'My briefcase was bursting at the seams,' he recalls. 'But carrying it was a bit of a physical workout for me, and I valued the exercise.'

Although he took a mountain of papers home, Michael still made dinnertime a priority and his family enjoyed lively conversations around the dining table. 'I loved hearing about my children's exploits and their views on life.' Always the diplomat, according to Jane, Michael steered dinner conversations away from party politics and instead centred on issues such as free speech, human rights and 'bigger picture topics'. Sometimes he mentioned his daily battles with hospital administrators, but Chris insists he didn't use the dinner table as a forum to vent his frustration. 'Dad didn't bring his anger home and was never outwardly furious. Even though we knew he had had a bad day at work, he remained even-keeled. He focused on the outcome of getting the best deal for his patients rather than worrying about being battered by terrible people. Dad was determined to either survive or outlive his opponents.'[64]

Jane recalls that after dinner Michael 'had a lovely way of redirecting us into doing the dishes'. While his children clattered around in the kitchen, he'd head for the study.[68] There he remained until eleven o'clock, reviewing the materials assembled by the working group and committees. 'It was painstaking and added to my exhaustion,' he recalls, 'but I knew it was a vital project, so I pushed on.' Michele often joined him there, doing the accounts for the patients Michael treated privately. Chris said his mum valiantly 'soldiered on' with clunky old software until a new accounting program became available.[64]

Because he believed pain medicine training was woefully inadequate, one of Michael's top priorities was educating doctors and allied health professionals. From early in his career, he had felt compelled to learn from the very best and he treasured the opportunity to learn from John Bonica, Patrick Wall and Ronald Melzack. 'The standards these three pioneers set became my benchmark and I longed for the next generation of doctors to embrace them,' he said. 'I felt a responsibility to share my knowledge and skills.'

Medical students receive little pain education, yet pain is the number one reason people go to the doctor. In 2018, 81,200 Australians visited their GP with a pain-related condition each day.[88] In the early 1990s, Laurie Mather raised the idea of introducing an interdisciplinary teaching program the team could take on the road, and for four years the pain centre's staff ran educational roadshows around New South Wales.[27] Later, when the former Flinders psychologist Professor Ross Harris joined the team, they developed this into a diploma and a master's degree in pain medicine at Sydney University.[26] The first twenty-eight students started in 1996, with the two-year part-time course attracting a diverse range of doctors and allied health professionals.

General practitioner, Dr Milana Votrubec, was in the first cohort of students to complete the Master in Pain Medicine. Michael's commitment to finding better ways of managing pain inspired Votrubec to do the same. She particularly valued the way he encouraged her to find answers to the many questions she raised.

'Think of the question, and then think about an action,' Michael would advise. 'Go and research it, because it will probably stick far better if you've looked it up yourself.'

Votrubec found it a refreshing way to learn compared to medical school where she had been 'taught by being told', soaking up information like a sponge rather than finding it out for herself.[89]

Professor Paul Glare, a palliative care physician, taught the program's cancer pain modules. 'I fondly remember spending Sunday mornings teaching on the fourth floor of the old chocolate brown building – a 'monolithic monstrosity' that was visible sticking up on the ridge from over the other side of Sydney Harbour – coaxing an ancient overhead projector to work,' he said. 'I was surprised that so many of the pain centre's team members happily gave up time on their weekends to teach.'[90]

Michael often gave lectures to the master's students and his son Chris would watch him rehearse before the weekend classes. 'Dad would have two slide carousels so he could put an image on one screen and his teaching materials on the other screen. I think it's an example of how he would go to the nth degree to make sure complicated concepts were translatable and easy to understand. He nurtured his students and would go to the earth's ends to help other people learn about pain medicine.'[64]

Sydney University initially offered the postgraduate programs to locals, then later to international students as online courses and through several universities overseas.

Michele and Michael still loved bushwalking although they didn't have much time to go on long walks. But the twins recall scenic hikes through Ku-ring-gai National Park and from Spit Bridge to Manly. Occasionally they visited the heritage-listed Blue Mountains, where they trekked at Govetts Leap, with its sandstone escarpments, sheer cliffs and thundering waterfalls. 'We would march in single file down fire trails deep into the Grose Valley,' Michael recalls. 'I loved smelling the eucalypts in Blue Gum Forest and seeing so many kookaburras and lizards. It felt a million miles away from my daily struggles at work.'

By now, the unstoppable Michael was also sharing his knowledge about pain medicine by giving orations in Australia and overseas. Michele said the audiences appreciated Michael's presentation style—informal and warm with everyday language rather than jargon—'very much his natural way of speaking'.[5] One year the European Society of Regional Anaesthesia invited him to deliver its annual address. He felt honoured. 'It was a tremendous opportunity to urge my colleagues to study the transition from acute to chronic pain and ways of preventing it.' Michele accompanied Michael to Barcelona for the lecture, which took place in a stiflingly hot auditorium. They enjoyed exploring the unique Spanish city.

During the lecture, Michael told the delegates that by the late 1980s many surgical wards had introduced acute pain teams to manage patients' pain after surgery.[91] 'Some of these teams used patient-controlled analgesia devices,' he explained to the audience of anaesthetists and pain researchers. 'They also injected epidural infusions of local anaesthetic and opioid mixtures. Still, despite these improvements, rates of uncontrolled pain after surgery remain far too high.'

Michael admitted one-third of his hospital's patients complained of severe pain at rest after surgery, despite the well-organised acute pain team. 'When we assessed patients presenting to our pain clinic with chronic pain, fourteen percent believed previous surgery was the initiating factor.' Michael shared his experiences of integrating pain services at Royal North Shore Hospital. 'Pain after surgery, cancer pain and chronic conditions such as low back pain are all managed within the same unit,' he said. 'Patients with cancer pain benefit from integrated pain services because they can access techniques normally used in acute and chronic pain management.'[91]

Towards the end of the lecture, Michael explained that pain specialists no longer regarded pain as a simple physiological activity but a complex dynamic condition. Pointing to the future, he urged his colleagues to place more emphasis on identifying patients at higher risk of developing chronic pain syndromes. He emphasised the importance of providing effective pain management after an operation. 'Failing to relieve pain is morally, ethically and economically unacceptable. It's up to us to solve this issue,' he insisted.[91]

During his presentation, Michael described several risk factors underpinning the transition from acute to chronic pain—the severity of the original pain, repeat surgery and anxiety before the operation, to name a few. 'The best way to reduce these risk factors is coordinated management by a team of surgeons, anaesthetists, psychologists and other health care professionals,' he argued.[91]

Michael encouraged his colleagues to focus on the crucial window of opportunity when acute pain progresses to persistent pain. 'It's vital to intervene during this transition phase,' he told them. Outlining the benefits of integrating services for managing acute, chronic and cancer pain, he noted that hospitals usually treat the distinct types of pain in separate facilities, using different medical and nursing teams. He carefully laid out the benefits of integration: the higher likelihood of detecting early signs of transition to chronic pain, and increased economic efficiencies because of shared resources.

'True integration of pain services requires large-scale institutional change,' Michael warned. 'Tragically, turf wars between departments, teams and professionals will slow the pace of this shift. We must act now to promote integration. It's up to us.'[91]

After the conference Michael and Michele headed to Portugal for five days. Once they arrived in Lisbon, they hired a car then drove up the coast, almost to Oporto. They stayed in a little ancient town and walked around the crumbling castle ramparts, feeling like they were living in the nineteenth century.

In 1996, much to his relief, Michael recruited Helen Johnston as his assistant. The pair forged a successful twenty-year partnership that saw Johnston, among her many other duties, type the manuscripts for several textbooks and dozens of speeches and journal articles.[92] Most nights after dinner, Michael dictated the content into an ancient Dictaphone, and the next day Johnston would type from the recordings. She worked diligently, rarely leaving the hospital before seven o'clock each evening. Michael appreciated her support immensely. 'Helen was a stalwart, enabling me to keep up a ninety-hour week at the hospital.' After finishing the evening's work with Johnston, Michael would sometimes head to the ballet or a concert at Sydney Opera House with Michele.

Life remained busy in the Cousins household as Jonathan and the twins travelled through their teenage years. James returned home for six months to study, delighting his parents and siblings. Michael and Michele both believed it was important for their children to participate in team sports to learn leadership and collaborative skills. They dedicated many weekends to cheering Jane from the sidelines when she played hockey, and as a proud 'Shore Boy', Michael loved to watch Jonathan and Chris play rugby and row on the team of his old school, Sydney Church of England Grammar School. Michael encouraged his children's sporting endeavours, and always proclaimed the importance of physical exercise. 'Dad would give us some advice,' Chris recalls, 'but ultimately, he wasn't trying to achieve anything through his kids, which is terrific.' Chris often noticed how 'measured, level-headed and straightforward' his father was when other parents were 'hurling abuse at the referee or yelling instructions to their sons from the sidelines'.[64]

Some weekends, Michael would help Jane prepare for her debating competitions. 'Dad loved quotations; he couldn't get enough of them, so we got stuck into a book of quotations together. His witty sense of humour often helped me shape my arguments, and he was always happy to listen while I practised my speeches.'[68]

On top of his hospital commitments, Michael kept up a heavy schedule of speeches on pain medicine both in Australia and overseas. One year, he felt honoured when the American Society of Anaesthesiologists invited him to present its annual oration in San Diego. With Michele in the audience, Michael decided to 'go out on a limb in his address', introducing two new concepts—pain relief as a universal human right and chronic pain as a disease in its own right. At the beginning of the lecture, he recounted a chilling description of chronic pain written by the psychologist LeShan:

Terrible things being done, worse threatened.
Outside forces in control. Will is helpless.
No time limit set. Cannot predict when it will end.
Pain is alien and meaningless. Consciousness turned inward.
Time perspective lost. Relationships weakened.[93]

Inviting the audience to 'climb into the skin' of a patient with severe unrelenting pain, Michael asked the delegates, mainly anaesthetists, 'What does LeShan's account of chronic pain suggest to you?' Then he effectively answered his own question: 'We must improve the way we treat chronic pain and change medical attitudes towards it.'

Lamenting the lack of government focus on chronic pain and its unacceptable human and economic costs, Michael passionately argued that societal attitudes towards people with chronic pain must change.

'Chronic pain is the silent epidemic,' he insisted. 'Patients with chronic pain often suffer silently. Relatives and others are silent; they hope it won't happen to them. Society is silent; mostly, it's unaware of the enormous human and financial cost. Politicians are silent because the costs are overwhelming. A huge gap exists between knowledge and practice, and this gap is widening as knowledge increases exponentially. Chronic pain will be regarded as the disease of the twenty-first century.'

Michael concluded his lecture by declaring: 'The plight of patients with chronic pain points to the need for a unique approach, one viewing pain relief as a basic human right. Everyone has a right to access pain management services.'

Asserting that it was up to pain professionals to take this concept to the community at large, Michael warned his audience it would be a tough call to change medical and societal attitudes. To some audience members, equating pain management with human rights was provocative and Michael's claim raised their hackles. A few anaesthetists urged him to 'tone down his comments'; they believed he was giving pain and its management too much prominence. 'They didn't want it to be so visible,' Michael explains. But refusing to be silenced, he encouraged his colleagues to take the lead in the larger debate that pain management was a fundamental human right. 'We would want nothing less for ourselves and certainly for our loved ones,' he added, lowering his voice for effect.

The second theme of Michael's lecture was one John Bonica had first proposed back in 1953 in his textbook on pain: chronic pain as a disease in its own right. Michael carefully laid out the emerging evidence that chronic pain could cause persistent physical effects within the nervous system: 'Pain receptors in the body can become sensitised by surgery or trauma, increasing the body's response to any noxious stimulus in the area of the pain.'[93]

This was the beginning of his crusade to have chronic pain recognised as a chronic disease. 'My claim was an explicit challenge to the prevailing orthodoxy that pain was merely a symptom of an underlying injury or illness. It was a controversial position to take and divided the pain medicine community.' Unperturbed, he persisted in the face of strident criticism from some of his colleagues.

Such criticism wasn't new to him. Throughout the 1990s, Michael had felt increasingly 'run down' by the relentless demands on his time and his frequent battles with the hospital's managers about funding and pain centre facilities. He left home at six-thirty each morning, even earlier on the days he implanted morphine pumps or did other surgical procedures on his patients. He rarely arrived home in the evening before seven o'clock and after dinner always headed to his study for several more hours of work.

One weekend some of Michael's friends at Palm Beach Surf Club encouraged him to take up the surf ski. The following weekend, he bought one and started training with his friends. Within a year he had mastered the sport, even in monstrous surf, and he competed in friendly surf club competitions. Michael believes this sport gave him a 'second lease of life' and was a 'godsend'. It also provided an outlet for him to 'tune out' from his worries.

One of the things that worried Michael was the lack of space at the pain centre. The enormous unmet demand for pain management services and the pain centre's rapidly growing research and educational initiatives strained the existing facilities, prompting Michael to ask the appeal board to raise more funds. Once again the community rallied, and the appeal board raised $6 million.

'It came down to the public, rather than governments, to identify pain management as a priority area and to build an integrated pain centre,' Michael sighed.

The new funds led to the centre's phase two development, made possible by the principal sponsorship of Manufacturers Mutual Insurance to the tune of $1.5 million each year for four years.[94]

Another of Michael's concerns was pain medicine training. For many years, he had urged the Melbourne-based Australian and New Zealand College of Anaesthetists, which trained specialist anaesthetists, to set up a pain medicine training program. Much to his delight, in the mid-1990s the college introduced a certificate in pain management for anaesthetists.[95] This program had similar content to the diploma and master's courses Michael had introduced at Sydney University, but anaesthetists across Australia and New Zealand could enrol in it because it didn't depend on them living in Sydney. Shortly afterwards, Michael contacted the leaders of five specialist medical colleges – representing anaesthetists, surgeons, physicians, psychiatrists and rehabilitation specialists – to suggest they form a Joint Advisory Committee on Pain Medicine.[95]

'To my surprise, they all agreed, and we soon started our work,' he recalls. 'I wanted to create a joint pain management training program for medical specialists.'

But it would be a torturous process, as he well understood. 'I knew trying to bring several medical specialties together to create a joint training program was a tough ask,' he admits, 'because of professional jealousies, vested interests and historic turf wars.'

Still, he pressed ahead, and during the following months, the concept gradually gained traction.[96] Fortunately, Michael was well-connected and knew several senior people within each medical college. He also had a 'secret weapon'.

'I kept a file card with the name and mobile phone number of the people heading each specialist college,' he grinned. 'It sat on the dashboard of my car. Every night while driving home, I would call the college leaders, working down the list then back around again'.

He kept talking to the college leaders about what he was doing, telling them he would continue to inform them about developments as they unfolded. 'I urged them to put aside their differences and to focus on broader objectives—improving pain medicine treatment, education and training.'

In March 1998, after months of intense debate, the two committees Michael chaired at the college of anaesthetists unanimously agreed to set up a Faculty of Pain Medicine to administer a single training and accreditation process for pain specialists. The involvement of five specialist colleges was in keeping with the interdisciplinary nature of pain management services. The committees submitted a proposal to the college of anaesthetists' leaders for approval.[95]

Over these years, Michael crusaded to convince the scientific and medical worlds that pain relief was a fundamental human right. 'I had a hunch that the more medical professionals and scientists acknowledged the human rights angle as a valid concept, the more it would appear to be a unanimous opinion from medical experts,' he recalls. 'Once it gained currency, I knew the next step was to garner the support of prominent members of the community—in philosophy, arts, lawmakers and legislators.' Michael hoped community leaders would pick up on the idea, put their weight behind it and discuss it persuasively within their circles and the mainstream media.

'As the concept built up a head of steam in society and the media, I thought it would place pressure on governments to prioritise pain management and fund it at the required level. I knew it was an ambitious long-term goal, but I was determined to put my plan into action.'

Meanwhile, during the 1990s, several studies highlighted the issue of increased prescribing of opioids for chronic pain. This was a controversial practice at the time and remains so today, with the USA[97] and some other Western nations, including Australia, struggling with an opioid epidemic.[98] In the late 1990s, the addiction medicine specialist, Dr James Bell, reported in the *Medical Journal of Australia* a seventy-three percent increase in the number of authorisations to prescribe opioids for chronic pain had occurred in the previous six years in New South Wales.[99] In an editorial in the same edition of the *Medical Journal of Australia*, Michael Cousins, Michael Nicholas and Allan Molloy also reported alarming statistics.[100] They revealed that prescribing of combined paracetamol-codeine had escalated from 1.9 million prescriptions at the beginning of the decade to 3.7 million five years later.

'Panadeine Forte was the second most prescribed drug in Australia,' Michael said. 'We argued that patients would achieve better outcomes, and governments would make considerable savings, if they invested more resources in interdisciplinary pain management services. We also recommended training to upskill GPs and medical specialists, so they referred patients with chronic pain to a specialised pain service rather than prescribing opioids.'

Tragically, their pleas 'fell on deaf ears'. No-one in political circles heeded their call to invest in interdisciplinary pain management. 'We held grave fears for the consequences of their complacency and inaction,' Michael said. 'It made me more resolute than ever to step up my advocacy.'

13

BIRTH OF THE PAIN MANAGEMENT RESEARCH INSTITUTE

AS the end of the twentieth century approached, Michael reflected on the pain centre's achievements. He felt pleased its research had improved several areas of pain management—including spinal cord injury, cancer, acute and chronic pain—but he was impatient and longed to make deeper inroads into unravelling the puzzle of pain. The centre's ballooning budget continually worried him and despite his constant badgering, he couldn't wring the funds he needed from the hospital's administrators. After discussing his funding shortfalls with fellow councillors at the National Health and Medical Research Council, he decided to apply to the council to appoint the pain centre as a 'Centre of Excellence'. If successful, this would secure three years of generous funding and enable the centre to fast-track its research.

Applying to the research council involved a laborious process. It was painstaking work, with Michael and his team documenting all the centre's research activities and publications. 'It kept me locked away in my study at night and on weekends for months, but I felt hopeful and thought we had a good chance.' Fortunately, Michael was able to listen to his favourite classical composers while working, and he kept a mountain of Beethoven and Mozart CDs next to his desk. Once the team finished the submission, Helen Johnston posted it, and their anxious wait for news from the research council began.[101]

Meanwhile, Michael continued to drive the discussions about setting up a Faculty of Pain Medicine. The College of Anaesthetists' council met for a full day at the Melbourne Club to review the pain committee's proposal. By that stage, Michael 'had a few people on side, but not that many' so he didn't know if he had the numbers to get his proposal over the line. 'It was touch and go.'

During the meeting, Michael fielded several heated objections. One council member remarked: 'Well, it's all very well, but I think it should just go around a few more times to let it mature a bit.' But the president disagreed, and the council members trawled through the proposal 'line by line, page by page'. Much to Michael's surprise, at the end of a long and exhausting day, the council approved the proposal. He was ecstatic. 'It took good running shoes to get the Faculty of Pain Medicine off the ground,' he said. 'No-one thought we could do it.'[95]

The agreement to run a joint training program, examination and specialist qualification for medical specialists was unique anywhere in the medical world.[102] Michael and Dr Richard Walsh, the council's president, wrote to the presidents of the five specialist colleges, asking them to nominate a member for the faculty's board. Soon afterwards the board members conducted their first meeting by teleconference, and Michael accepted their invitation for him to serve as faculty dean. Michael was relieved the teleconference went so well because one week later he was due to travel to Boston for the wedding of his oldest son, James, and he didn't want to leave faculty matters 'up in the air' while he was in America for three weeks with his family.

Michael loved seeing his son, James, marry and his family holiday after the wedding energised him. But before he knew it his overseas trip was over and it was back to work. Despite the daily grind, he was excited because soon after returning from overseas the Faculty of Pain Medicine's board was due to have its first face-to-face meeting – on 4 February 1999.

'It was a historic day for pain medicine in Australia and New Zealand,' Michael wrote in the *ANZCA Bulletin* shortly after the meeting. 'It marked the beginning of specialist pain medicine training and heralded a unique level of professionalism in pain medicine.'[103]

Associate Professor Roger Goucke, a specialist pain medicine physician at the Sir Charles Gairdner Hospital in Perth, said everyone thought setting up the faculty was an excellent idea, 'but it seemed like an impossible dream'. Goucke believes launching the faculty was the only way Australia could advance pain medicine practice. 'Michael Cousins recognised that if the nation had a respectable, well-organised professional body, then pain would have a higher profile within medical circles and government,' he said.[104]

Goucke knew the specialist medical colleges in the United Kingdom wanted to set up a training organisation. But they struggled to do it because the colleges for surgeons, physicians and psychiatrists all wanted to 'do their own thing'. 'They felt that if they had to join, who would be the boss? Who would be the manager? Where was the money going to come from? Territorial battles and turf wars obstructed the process.'[104] The Royal College of Anaesthetists in England did set up a Faculty of Pain Medicine, but it wasn't until 2007—nine years after Australia and it only included anaesthetists.[105]

Looking back on those years, Associate Professor Carolyn Arnold, a pain medicine physician at Alfred Health in Victoria and the Australian Pain Society's first female president, believes most pain medicine professionals felt isolated before the faculty formed.

'The Faculty of Pain Medicine quickly brought everyone together,' she said. 'To some extent pain clinics were full of disappointed patients who had failed other treatments. Many doctors felt a sense of hopelessness about working in a pain clinic but establishing pain medicine as a specialty provided us, and our patients, with a higher profile. It also legitimised the field of pain medicine.'[106]

Professor Pam Macintyre, Director of the Acute Pain Service at Royal Adelaide Hospital and a member of the faculty's inaugural board, concurs, saying that before Michael set up the faculty, many in the pain medicine community were naysayers and thought it wouldn't work. She admits Michael did things single-mindedly, which put some people offside. 'Over the years Michael had his detractors who thought he was too big for his boots and self-promoting, but he was the one with the get-up-and-go; he got things going,' she said.[107]

As the new century approached, tennis continued to be one of Michael's favourite pastimes on busy weekends and long summer evenings. The Cousins family spent many happy hours playing doubles together and Michael was known for sneaking his racquet into his left hand to make the game a little more challenging. Before his regular Saturday afternoon tennis game with friends, Michael would meticulously sweep up the leaves on the court then sprinkle chlorine around the edges to prevent mould from growing there.

On the work front, after months of anxious waiting for a response from the research council, Michael was ecstatic when he received a letter informing him that the centre's application had been successful. It meant they could rely on three years of secure funding. 'The research council award boosted our morale and the centre's funding at a time of rapid growth,' he recalls.

Around the same time, the pain centre board renamed the research arm 'The Pain Management Research Institute' and the hospital named the pain clinic 'The Pain Management Research Centre'.

In July 1999, the research council's working party on acute pain finished writing its guideline on acute pain management and the Australian Government published *Acute Pain Management: Scientific Evidence*.[108] The guideline described the causes of acute pain and offered health professionals advice on how to assess and treat a myriad of painful conditions such as burns and pain after surgery. It also provided guidance on acute pain management in children and patients with special needs, such as those from non-English speaking backgrounds. This document would become a watershed resource internationally.

The guideline attracted an avalanche of media coverage, and as the spokesperson for the working party, Michael was run off his feet doing interviews. Fortunately, by then he had taken part in professional media training in a set-up that mimicked a television studio. He felt the training had 'systematised' his technique and reinforced the things he did well in an interview. 'It helped a lot to fine-tune my skills.'

Michael found it challenging to fit media commentary into his work schedule because he meticulously prepared for each interview. Still, he believed media coverage was essential to improving government and public awareness of pain and its proper management. He told journalists pain management was a fundamental human right, and medical professionals must properly treat acute pain to prevent it transitioning to chronic pain. 'Most people incorrectly assume severe pain is something patients must endure, and it's an inevitable consequence of an illness, injury or operation. I'm determined to change this view.' [109] [110] [111]

As well as educating the general public about pain, Michael wanted his media commentary to reduce the stigma associated with chronic pain. In his interviews, he said: 'People with chronic pain fear others will perceive them as a malingerer or hypochondriac. It's a silent epidemic because the people who live with chronic pain day after day, year after year are too afraid to speak about it.'[110]

A few months later, Michael updated his college of anaesthetist colleagues on the Faculty of Pain Medicine's progress. In the college's newsletter, *ANZCA Bulletin*, he wrote that several pain centres around Australia had applied for accreditation as approved training centres for pain specialists. He noted that when the faculty reviewed the pain centres, hospital administrators often corrected the deficiencies immediately to ensure the faculty accredited its pain centre. In the update, Michael thanked the board for its tremendous work and concluded that the Faculty of Pain Medicine had achieved much in 1999—the first year of its existence.[101]

Several talented pain specialists joined the Pain Management Research Centre team because of its integrated scientific research and patient treatment. The paediatric pain specialist, Dr Suellen Walker, valued the opportunity to combine patient treatment in the pain clinic and scientific experiments in the institute's laboratory.[112] She felt privileged to have the chance to link her laboratory studies and clinical care and be able to take clinical questions back to the lab, and vice versa.

Professor Chris Vaughan, who now heads the basic research department, agrees. He appreciated how Michael encouraged the basic scientists to visit the pain clinic and listen to patients to help them understand the nature of pain problems. Hearing patients speak about their experiences helped Vaughan better understand pain and led him to change his research focus to studying nerve pain. He also learned an incredible amount by participating in the pain clinic ward rounds, 'because Michael had such a good understanding of what was causing each patient's pain, and he could explain it in layman's language to them'.[113]

Suellen Walker also enrolled in the centre's master's degree. She appreciated how the course brought together professionals from across several disciplines because they could share their differing viewpoints. Walker was also impressed that so many overseas doctors travelled to Sydney to study with Michael.[112] Many of them returned home to be trailblazers, and within a few years, graduates of the centre's postgraduate programs took up leadership positions in pain centres around the world.

During these years Michele always invited the pain medicine trainees home for lunches and whenever one of Michael's overseas colleagues such as John Loeser or Dan Carr visited Australia for a conference, they stayed with the Cousins. Carr admired the way Michele's unwavering support contributed to Michael's success. 'There was an interval,' Carr said, 'when Michael probably spent more time on aeroplanes than on the ground. Michele held it all together. She is a very gracious lady.'[39] Marc Russo agrees. 'With his wife, Michele, they have been a formidable team.'[72]

Many of Michael's colleagues agreed he could take on so much not only because of Michele's backing but also because he was adept at managing teams of highly skilled professionals. Laurie Mather recalls Michael had a reputation for 'being a superb judge of people's skills and capacity and putting the right people in the right job'. Michael appointed highly accomplished people to senior positions, delegating challenging projects to them and empowering them to get the job done. 'He was good at inspiring people to achieve things they never thought they could accomplish,' Mather said. 'Michael led by example, had enormous expectations and got the best out of people, but some colleagues found him far too demanding.'[27]

Philip Siddall said Michael was continually searching for talented people and if he thought a team member was on board and committed, he invested time and energy in mentoring them. However, Siddall believes Michael could be conflict-averse when it came to addressing interpersonal conflict between team members. 'He sometimes let things go rather than confronting an underperforming employee or resolving conflict between team members.' But when the conflict involved administrative roadblocks and hurdles or something he wanted to achieve for the pain centre, Michael wouldn't step back. 'He would charge straight ahead or go around the obstacle,' Siddall said. [73]

By the end of the century, the international pain medicine community regarded the pain centre as a world leader in research and patient treatment.[21] [39] [20] But Michael often felt 'at his wit's end' with the chronic underfunding and believed mismanagement was rife at the hospital. He and some of the other department heads thought one of the major problems was a lack of delegated decision-making—this meant that Michael and his senior colleagues couldn't make staffing and equipment decisions without consulting officers at a higher level of the health bureaucracy than the hospital's senior managers. Staff morale at Royal North Shore Hospital was steadily dwindling, which saddened Michael. But it strengthened his resolve to step up his fundraising efforts to ensure he could continue to support the pain centre's team and maintain their optimism and passion.

The year 1999 was pivotal for the Cousins. Michael celebrated his sixtieth birthday and thirty-five years since he had decided to specialise in pain medicine. Jane and Chris Cousins also completed their last year of school. One incident that year deeply affected Chris and he said it reflected his father's approach to life. It was the eve of his final 'Head of the River' rowing regatta, and Shore's tradition was to hold a 'Telegram Night' at its boatshed. Rather than faxing the usual rallying cry or 'win at all costs' type of message, Michael had sent Rudyard Kipling's poem *If*.[114] Kipling wrote the poem as paternal advice to his young son. Chris felt the poem typified his father's 'gentlemanly approach to sportsmanship', in that he encouraged him to give the race 'every last ounce of energy and sinew', rather than insisting he must try to win.[64]

Meanwhile Michael continued spending nights and weekends writing grant applications. It was laborious and time-consuming, and he resented how it soaked up so much of his leisure time. Still, he and his colleagues accepted it was a vital part of sustaining academic endeavours. Over the years they were often successful, attracting enough funding to finance many research studies. But they also had their share of bitter disappointments, missing out on securing some competitive research grants. While grants from corporate entities contributed some funding, they didn't provide the recurrent funding required to run an interdisciplinary pain centre on a sustainable footing. And Michael worried about the potential for a conflict of interest when pharmaceutical and medical devices companies provided support; he didn't want to have to depend on them too much.

Brian Davidson, who chairs the Pain Management Research Institute's fundraising organisation, Pain Foundation, believes it is difficult to raise funds for pain research because of the intense competition for the charity dollar. Rather than trying to attract donations from the general public, the centre focused on building long-term relationships with donors. Davidson considers one of Michael's strengths during these years was his ability to 'open doors' for fundraising because of his high profile and knack of communicating a simple message to donors. As Davidson listened to Michael talking to people about the plight of patients with chronic pain, he noticed how the stories resonated with those in the room. 'Michael clearly explained to donors the lack of a quick fix to curing pain; instead, he told them it was a matter of helping patients through interdisciplinary pain management.'[115]

Roger Goucke claims that in the early days Michael was the only person in Australia to have the right personality and 'inexhaustible enthusiasm' needed to raise the enormous sums of money, personnel and real estate required to set up two world-class pain centres.[104] Dr Charles Brooker, who joined Royal North Shore Hospital's pain centre in the early 1990s, agrees. He admired Michael's fundraising ability but felt daunted by the sheer number of projects his mentor juggled. Brooker revealed that like many pioneers and leaders, Michael didn't dot the 'i's and cross the 't's. 'Instead, he came up with the idea, kickstarted the project, secured funding and surrounded himself with highly competent people who would look after the fine details.'[116]

Brooker appreciated the way Michael was so forward-thinking. 'He was always thinking ahead, focused on the next step and the next step after that. But this meant he was exhausting to work with, always setting the pace. Whenever the team had a small win, rather than celebrating, he had a habit of saying, "Oh, well, that's great, now what about this?"' Brooker recalls some colleagues felt Michael was leaving all the work to others, but most knew Michael was hard at it himself. 'He never complained about it.'

By the end of the twentieth century Michael felt immensely proud of the centre's achievements but impatient for it to keep making progress. He was relieved the team had advanced the treatment of pain on so many fronts and that these techniques were filtering through to clinical practice. He and his colleagues had helped thousands of patients live better lives, and he was determined to expand the clinic, despite the personal costs of combining vigorous fundraising with everything else he juggled. Still, he looked forward to the new millennium and mapped out ambitious plans to further advance the field of pain medicine in Australia.

14

THE 2000s

AS the new century dawned, Michael worried that pain management was still not on national agendas. Nor was it high in the awareness of Australia's state governments, which meant it was chronically underfunded.[117] At every opportunity, he urged politicians, bureaucrats and his hospital's administrators to focus on pain and its management. But they ignored his arguments, and some were openly hostile towards him. On top of this, he was deeply disappointed that most people in the general community misunderstood chronic pain. 'To some extent, chronic pain has a rather cruel and unfortunate label,' he explains. 'People with lower back pain are sometimes characterised in a very condescending manner, and this goes back a long way, even to cartoons in former eras.'

Although he knew it was essential to kickstart a community conversation, Michael recognised this wouldn't be a straightforward task. The linchpin, he thought, would be collecting data on the magnitude of the pain problem, then recruiting several high-profile individuals to talk about the issue.

Michael spoke with the Pain Management Research Institute's epidemiologist, Professor Fiona Blyth, about his idea. She shared his vision because of her growing understanding of chronic pain as a significant public health problem. They agreed Blyth would analyse data from health surveys to estimate the prevalence and cost of chronic pain. The pair knew they could use this information to educate both politicians and the public about pain.

Blyth based one of her first studies on data from the New South Wales Health Department's first state-wide adult health survey.[118] In this study, she evaluated over 17,000 responses, finding fifteen percent of men and twenty percent of women suffered from chronic pain. Armed with these statistics, Michael met with politicians and bureaucrats to encourage them to increase the funding of pain management services around Australia to meet soaring demand. Ever the agitator, he encouraged his colleagues to do the same.

During these demanding times one way Michael relaxed at night and on weekends was to watch Australia's national rugby union team, the Wallabies, competing. Jane recalls the only time she ever heard her father yelling was when he watched the Wallabies on television. 'Dad worshipped the Wallabies, and their winger, David Campese, was his hero.' Michael often took his family to see Wallabies matches, and according to Jane, he went 'all out' when the Rugby World Cup and Olympic Games were in Sydney, buying tickets to 'everything under the sun'.[68]

Meanwhile, the Faculty of Pain Medicine board continued to forge ahead, developing a curriculum to support training and accrediting several pain clinics throughout Australia and New Zealand. The faculty's education committee, under the leadership of Professor Milton Cohen AM, a specialist pain medicine physician and rheumatologist at Sydney's St Vincent's Hospital, took great strides. The curriculum was rigorous, preparing staff in pain centres to assess and treat the multiple aspects of pain. Education committee members also developed the structure for the first examination, and Michael said it delighted him that twelve candidates had applied to sit the exam.[119]

By July 2000, the faculty's inaugural board had completed its term. Michael thanked each member for the harmonious and effective way they had worked together. 'It is a tribute to the individuals who have worked on this board to quickly form a team approach that is so characteristic of interdisciplinary pain medicine,' he wrote in the *ANZCA Bulletin*.[120] Welcoming newly elected board members, he warned they faced some crucial challenges, including the creation of more training positions in interdisciplinary pain centres. 'Clearly, a major manpower shortage exists in this new specialty and representations will be made by the board to both federal and state governments,' he wrote.

Michael believed pain medicine would achieve greater prominence and priority if viewed as a specialist area of medical practice rather than as a subspecialty of anaesthesia. He suggested to the Faculty of Pain Medicine that it pair up with the Australian Pain Society to lobby the Australian Medical Council to recognise pain as a field of medicine in its own right. He set up a working party to plan a formal submission. After several meetings, the members decided it would be best for the faculty and pain society to create separate proposals, believing this would give more weight to their advocacy. The working party agreed the faculty submission would emphasise its unique role as a training and education body for five specialist medical colleges.[117]

Roger Goucke and Michael set to work to assemble the evidence required by the Australian Medical Council which, according to Goucke, entailed 'a comprehensive, in-depth, detailed proposal, including exhaustive specifics about the background of what the faculty was trying to do, what was going on in pain medicine around the world and how the faculty intended to grow'.[104] During this time, Michael and the college of anaesthetists' president met with the Federal Health Minister, Dr Michael Wooldridge, to inform him of the faculty's intention. They hoped he would understand why it was essential to professionalise pain medicine because the minister had previously admitted that chronic pain was one of the three most costly health conditions in Australia. To Michael's relief, the health minister agreed that pain was a neglected area of medicine and that professionalising it was an urgent priority.[121] But that was the easy step in the process.

Michael always wore a dark navy suit and immaculate white shirt to meetings, but he wasn't interested in clothes. Early in their marriage

Michele gave up on trying to get him to a tailor because it would involve three visits and Michael refused to waste so much time on buying clothes. So Michele bought his clothes. She would find a suit she liked, take it home for Michael to try on, then 'cart' it back to the shop to have the trouser hems taken up. 'To get him in there you'd have to get his arm up behind his back,' she said. 'He would sometimes go to the shops, but I had to push him. After two hours, he really badly wanted to get out of there. He was not about to go shopping voluntarily—ever! The other thing was he wanted to buy all the shoes and several suits at the same time. He just wanted to say "yes" to everything so he could get out and wouldn't have to return'.[5]

In 2002, after completing his three-year term, Michael stepped down as the Faculty of Pain Medicine Dean. By the time of his retirement from this position, the faculty truly represented an interdisciplinary approach to pain medicine. The new dean, Leigh Atkinson, was a neurosurgeon and the vice-dean, Milton Cohen, a rheumatologist. The examination committee chair, Dr Penny Briscoe, was an anaesthetist, and several psychiatrists and rehabilitation specialists served on the board and committees.[122]

Michael told his colleagues the faculty had made much progress since its inception but reminded them many challenges lay ahead. These included developing training posts in pain centres, increasing public awareness of chronic pain as a serious health care issue, and increasing pain medicine's profile. Reiterating the urgency of gaining recognition of pain as a specialist area of medicine, he said the faculty had already assembled much of the evidence the medical council had requested, but much more work lay ahead.[122]

In 2003 Michael and Michele bought an old house with a spectacular view of Palm Beach and Barrenjoey. They had dreamt about buying a holiday house there for the previous decade. It was a refuge for Michael, who at sixty-four still worked at his desk until late each night even though he felt intensely fatigued. By then he had published 208 papers, steadily logging a published paper every eight weeks for thirty-two years.[22] Even though Michael and Michele stayed at Palm Beach every weekend, Michael still spent the bulk of his time there 'holed up in the study'. However, he would always squeeze in some bodysurfing and a morning or two of paddling his beloved surf ski. Sometimes he played a game of golf or tennis and, when time permitted, he read biographies and the 'Classics' or played chess with Chris.

'It kept me sane,' Michael recalls. 'I just had to keep grinding away every weekend. You can do it, but you can't do it forever. In retrospect, it was too much. It took a big toll and left me depleted. My body and I burned out. Sooner or later, everything breaks.'

Michael dearly wanted to retire, and he continually primed colleagues to take on his job at Royal North Shore Hospital. But it was a tough job to go into. 'There were plenty of challenging issues to cope with and it was exhausting to deal with them. Whenever I thought one of my colleagues would accept the Chair in Pain Medicine, they ended up deciding against it. Instead, they went into private practice. Nobody could face it.'

In 2004 Michael started campaigning for medical professionals to view chronic pain as a disease in its own right. He knew it would affect how they managed chronic pain clinically. And he also had a hunch—it would profoundly influence the way governments and hospitals prioritised chronic pain for funding. In a paper Michael and Philip Siddall published in the journal, *Anesthesia and Analgesia,* they argued that chronic pain was a disease in its own right rather than a passive warning signal of an underlying disease process or tissue damage.[123] They outlined the evidence supporting the concept, proposing for chronic pain to qualify as a disease entity; it should have its own pathology, symptoms and signs rather than merely being a symptom of another disease process. They insisted chronic pain met the criteria for a disease entity and persistent pain gave rise to its own secondary pathology, a 'constellation of symptoms and signs indicative of persistent pain'. This position was controversial and polarised opinion among Australia's pain community. Michael faced intense criticism from some of his colleagues, but he forged ahead, determined to convince them of his argument's veracity.

A few pain physicians who wish to remain anonymous believe classifying chronic pain as a disease forces people with chronic pain into a disease model, undermining treatment approaches focused on empowering patients to self-manage their pain. They also say the disease model further increases the stigmatisation of people with chronic pain. But Michael considered classifying chronic pain as a disease would enhance its assessment and attract more attention and funding from governments for improved treatment.[124]

Philip Siddall said viewing chronic pain as a disease entity is more than a physiological or clinical issue. 'It's also a political issue because the medical profession has always viewed chronic pain as a symptom of an underlying condition. The outcome of viewing pain as a disease is crucial because it means the health system treats it differently, and it attracts more recognition and resources.'[73]

Roger Goucke believes the debate around classifying chronic pain as a disease is a matter of semantics.[104] While he thinks such a classification is an excellent idea, he acknowledges some people don't accept it. He has seen hundreds of patients during his career and claims that while they may have started with a fractured ankle or prolapsed vertebral disc, 'they have ended up with chronic pain, and this pain is their problem rather than the initial injury'. He supports the idea of chronic pain as a disease because of the central nervous system changes that cause persistent pain. 'So the answer is no more surgery,' Goucke insists. 'Surgery won't fix the problem because the issue presenting now is a central nervous system malfunction. If you accept that pain can be freestanding, it lets you focus on the pain and actually focus on managing the pain, rather than doing more and more investigations, more and more tests and more and more operations.'[104]

Meanwhile, in 2004 Dr Brenda Lau was completing her anaesthesia training at the University of British Columbia, and in her last year, she studied chronic pain. It intrigued her, so she hunted around the world for an accredited training program that would give her a fellowship in pain medicine. She came to Australia knowing, 'Michael Cousins ran the best accredited training program in the world'.[125]

Lau 'loved every minute of the program', and after qualifying as a pain medicine specialist, she told Michael she planned to remain in Australia for another year. She was keen to study health economics because she wanted to learn about the systems and policies shaping whether health services such as pain clinics would continue to grow or wither and die. Lau's goal was to learn ways of influencing interdisciplinary pain management in her home country because she worried about the sustainability of pain clinics there. When she left Canada, few pain clinics existed, and the country lacked a nationally coordinated interdisciplinary pain management system. She wanted to return to her homeland and improve the outlook for Canadians suffering with chronic pain.

At first, Lau's decision surprised Michael. He thought she would be eager to return to Canada, but he admired her passion for pain medicine because it matched his own. He offered to act as her supervisor while she completed a master's degree in medicine at Sydney University. The pair met every Friday afternoon for a long chat about pain medicine and its future. Lau cherished these conversations and appreciated the time Michael spent with her. 'He was extremely busy but also a patient man who thoroughly enjoyed sharing his knowledge,' she said. 'I think we had a unique relationship because I love pain medicine so much.'[125]

Michael and Roger Goucke continued to compile the mountain of documents required by the Australian Medical Council. It took them several years, but to their great relief, in 2005 the council agreed to recognise pain medicine as a specialty. This recognition was a pivotal moment for the profession. It meant pain medicine physicians could bill at specialist rates, encouraging more doctors to become pain specialists and many more patients to access pain management services. It was a significant milestone in the growing reputation of the Faculty of Pain Medicine. It also illustrated the federal government's acceptance of pain medicine as a medical specialty in its own right.[102]

Milton Cohen considers that gaining this specialty recognition was a crucial step forward because beforehand, pain and its treatment had always been such a low priority. 'Pain was only ever a symptom of something else, not a problem in its own right,' he said. 'When you applied the usual rules of Western medicine, too many people didn't get better. Cohen admits there's an argument that pain medicine doesn't need to be a specialty because the management of pain should be within the compass of all medical graduates.

'But the reality is it's not,' he said, 'because pain is neglected and such a complex area'.[126]

Roger Goucke agrees. He maintains that once Australia secured recognition of pain medicine as a specialty, Europe followed, and so did the Irish. 'It was just waiting for someone to crystallise the thinking,' he says.[104]

Goucke explains that after the Faculty of Pain Medicine formed and the federal government recognised the specialty, Medicare accepted item numbers for pain specialists. But it took a tremendous amount of lobbying to achieve this outcome. 'Before the change, if anaesthetists provided pain management services, the item numbers they used didn't cover the cost of the lengthy consultations,' Goucke explains. 'So it disadvantaged them because the item numbers for anaesthetists were for procedures rather than the extended consultations required for pain management.'[104]

In the meantime, during the first of their Friday afternoon conversations, Lau and Michael discussed the history of interdisciplinary pain management. Over the following weeks and months, they progressed to present-day challenges in pain medicine—both local and global.

Sometimes on weekends, Michael and Michele invited the pain medicine fellows to join them at Palm Beach. 'Despite Michael and Michele having achieved so much for so many, on a personal level, they were grounded, laid-back, incredibly warm and welcoming to their staff, colleagues and fellows,' Lau recalls. 'Michael's favourite past-time was surf skiing and the water. To get to know this side of Michael with his family was heartwarming.' Lau remembers these visits fondly because every moment is a 'teaching moment' for Michael. 'As much is learned about pain medicine on the water as it is on the hospital wards—patience, agility, problem-solving, pattern recognition and intuition,' she jests.[125]

Another memorable event in Michael's life happened in 2005—Jane married her American fiancé, Charlie Kuehn, in the chapel at Michael's old school. As Michael walked down the aisle with his beloved daughter, his eyes filled with tears.[68] It was a bittersweet moment for him because he knew the following morning Jane would leave to live in America.

Meanwhile, Fiona Blyth's PhD research had included an analysis of the societal and personal costs of chronic pain, including the effects of pain on work performance, levels of disability, and use of pain-relieving drugs and health services. In the first study in Australia, and one of a few worldwide, Blyth documented total lost workdays and associated annual costs because of the disease. Her study was the first to show lower levels of disability in people using active self-management strategies such as paced exercise and cognitive behavioural therapy.[127-129]

In 2007 Blyth chaired the steering committee for an Access Economics study, *The High Price of Pain*.[130] Access Economics estimated chronic pain cost the Australian economy $34 billion per annum, making it the nation's third most costly health problem. As the study leader, Michael acted as media spokesperson. He told journalists the results should prompt action to prevent pain from going untreated.

'It's now possible to manage persistent pain in seventy to eighty percent of patients,' he said in one interview, 'yet fewer than ten percent of people obtain pain relief. Federal and state governments could save enormous amounts of public funds by providing the resources to deliver proper treatment. At least half of the patients who access effective treatment get back to a reasonable lifestyle, offering savings on hospital and doctor visits, x-rays, surgery, medications and productivity.'[131]

Fiona Blyth's research has been integral to educating politicians, policymakers and the general public about chronic pain's personal and societal costs. It has also underpinned health policy reform. Reflecting on the impact of her research, Blyth maintains it has given pain a 'shape' because it reveals the size of the problem for the community.

'It showed chronic pain was highly prevalent and was more common than several other well-known conditions,' she said.[132]

When speaking with patients and community groups, Blyth noticed people living with pain expressed surprise when she revealed the condition's prevalence. 'For the first time, they realised they were not alone, and chronic pain was a common problem. It wasn't something I had planned as an impact of the work,' she admits, 'but it's personally important to me that my research has given people living with pain a sense of comfort to know they weren't suffering on their own'.[132]

The year 2007 was significant for Michael's family too, with James Cousins competing in the elite Ironman triathlon in Kailua-Kona, in the western part of Hawaii. Michael, Michele and Jonathan flew from Australia to cheer him on while he swam, cycled and ran in the scorching heat. They rented a large house and Jane and Charlie joined them there.

Shortly after arriving home from Hawaii, Michael became aware that Royal North Shore Hospital planned to build a new campus. He felt excited because it would mean he may be able to expand the pain clinic, which treated thousands of patients each year and struggled to meet escalating demand because of a lack of space. But to his dismay, he soon learned the hospital's plans didn't include a pain centre. Aghast, he couldn't believe the administrators had excluded a pain clinic when the demand for pain services was so strong. Michael believed several forces were at play—cost-cutting, historic turf wars, tall poppy syndrome and professional jealousy. He knew fighting for the pain centre would be an uphill battle and a monumental test, but he resolved to get the best deal for pain patients.

Michael arranged an urgent meeting with the hospital's administrators. He took Charles Brooker, now head of the hospital's pain management department, with him. On the way, Michael told Brooker how he had worked as a porter at the hospital while studying medicine and it was during that time he had his first taste of dealing with hospital administrators. 'It all started back then,' he grinned as he asked Brooker to tread on his toes under the table if he became too fired up during the meeting. When they reached the designated room, they sat on one side of a large boardroom table. Three hospital managers dressed in dark suits sat on the other side. Michael felt as if he could 'cut the air with a knife' because the atmosphere was so tense.

The meeting started with a senior manager explaining the hospital used a 'patient-centred care model' to determine funding priorities. Michael and Brooker glanced at each other, knowing the model would leave their pain patients with nothing.

Michael stood up, noisily pushing back his chair. 'Thanks for outlining all this. The model we established for multidisciplinary care is well accepted around the world and we raised considerable community and government support to build the current centre. I'm sure you'll agree we're setting a high standard of care for patients with this model. So we just need to know where the centre is going to be located...?' He returned to his seat but continued to push the point, dominating the meeting so it couldn't move on. Occasionally, he 'just let it fly'.[116]

Afterwards, as they sprinted back to the pain clinic—Michael with sore toes—Brooker asked Michael for some tips on negotiating. The response astounded him. 'Discuss nothing specific at a meeting,' Michael advised. 'Try to come out of it without agreeing to anything, then negotiate in the background later.' Michael explained that his approach was to arrive ready to confirm an agreement he had already negotiated because he believed it was impossible to get a controversial topic sorted out in your favour in a meeting. 'Ensure you nail down everything before a meeting. If you haven't settled an agreement beforehand, it's best to go in and grit your teeth and get out conceding nothing,' he added.[116]

Meanwhile, Michael and Brenda Lau continued their Friday afternoon conversations and in 2008, Lau wrote her thesis, *Change or Die: The Future of Multidisciplinary Pain Centers*.[133] In her conclusions, she emphasised that pain medicine professionals needed to play an active role in shaping health care systems. Otherwise, interdisciplinary pain centres risked being eliminated because they are so resource intensive. She cited the situation in the USA, where after flourishing in the 1980s, pain clinics dwindled to a handful because health insurance companies refused to pay for interdisciplinary pain services. 'Insurance companies considered these services too expensive, preferring to fund one-off procedures such as nerve blocks and spinal stimulators rather than interdisciplinary pain management, which is the only gold standard of complex chronic pain management.'[125]

On the home front, Michael continued to treasure his weekends at the beach. His family's holiday house provided an escape from his constant battles about the hospital's redevelopment plans. It also acted as a natural meeting place for his adult children, grandchildren, friends, Geoff Cousins and Pam who all frequently gathered there. James Cousins had moved to Brisbane in the meantime, but he and his family always stayed with Michael and Michele for the Christmas holidays, and Jane and Charlie often flew across from America to join them. Michael loved it. 'Having his family around him is the most important thing for Dad,' Jane said. 'He is at his happiest when we sit around the house talking or go down to the beach. For him just being with us is what brings him joy.'[68]

In March 2008, the New South Wales Government conducted the Garling inquiry into the state's health system following a series of high-profile medical mishaps in hospitals, including at Royal North Shore. Michael and several of his demoralised colleagues gave evidence. He told the commissioner he had watched staff morale and hospital standards erode in the past decade.

'After fifty years of observing this hospital, I'm sad to say over the last ten to twelve years, there has been an erosion. I'm on a knife-edge,' he said, adding that he and fellow senior staff were seriously considering resigning.[134]

Michael also told the inquiry that funding promised by the New South Wales Government in 2002 was still outstanding despite the pain centre becoming a state-wide service with a more extensive remit. He said most of the pain management centres operating in Australia's hospitals were based on his designs, and yet his own hospital had not consulted him over its redevelopment plans. Despite his repeated attempts to improve the pain centre's funding, the New South Wales Government continued to claim the centre had adequate funds.

'It really concerns me to hear there is not agreement that we are underfunded,' he added.[134]

In the inquiry's final report, the commissioner wrote: 'During the course of this inquiry, I have identified one impediment to good, safe care which infects the whole public hospital system. I liken it to the Great Schism of 1054.[iv] It is the breakdown of good working relations between clinicians and management, which is detrimental to patients. It is alienating the most skilled in the medical workforce from service in the public system. If it continues, New South Wales will risk losing one of the crown jewels of its public hospital system: the engagement of the best and brightest from the professions who are able to provide world-class care in public hospitals free of charge to the patient.'[135]

Throughout the following months, Michael and Brooker took part in several heated meetings about the hospital's redevelopment plans. But they despaired of gaining the space they needed. Brooker admired the way his mentor operated during this exasperating process. 'Whenever Michael couldn't achieve an acceptable outcome,' Brooker said, 'he went over people's heads and rang someone more senior. He wasn't afraid to go around people, to a point where the person he was talking to might be a little surprised he had gone above them, but they would admire his audacity.' Once in front of a senior person, Michael would offer them 'an eminently reasonable' arrangement. 'I think we can achieve this,' he would say. 'It'll be a little bit of cost here, but we can make it back, and the benefits will be X, Y and Z'.[116]

Brooker noticed that Michael always had a game plan worked out in advance. Despite his intense frustration, Michael never lost his cool and was always polite but doggedly persisted until he had achieved the outcome he sought. When something didn't go his way, he kept driving forward and brushed off disappointments. Struggling through some challenging times, Michael just gritted his teeth and marched on until he had accomplished whatever he was trying to achieve. According to Brooker, Michael wasn't affected by other people's opinions of him, which probably helped him survive many turbulent months of hostile meetings.[116]

In late 2008, the Pain Management Research Institute's board recruited a former pharmacist and public relations consultant, Lesley Brydon. Board members wanted Brydon to increase awareness of PMRI's research on the value of interdisciplinary pain management and to help raise funds for the centre's ambitious research program.

Brydon created a briefing pack for journalists about PMRI and its research programs, issued a media release, then organised a round of TV, print and radio interviews for Michael. The response astonished her. In the days following the publicity, the pain clinic's phone 'rang off the hook' as people desperate for help telephoned. The callers came from around

Australia, revealing a widespread, unmet need for pain services, especially in regional, rural and remote areas. The response prompted Brydon to wonder what was happening in pain clinics elsewhere in the country.

In the following months, she contacted the registered pain clinics in each state and was concerned by what she discovered. 'There were fifteen pain clinics, all in major cities, but no two of them offered the same programs,' she recalls. While all pain clinics in public hospitals were led by pain specialists, the composition of their interdisciplinary teams varied, and the services offered at each depended on the skills available. 'Most clinics had a psychologist and a physiotherapist but the programs at each differed widely. No other clinic offered an intensive three-week pain management program such as ADAPT. If they offered a structured program, its scope was limited because of capacity, skill or resource constraints.'[136]

The lack of best practice interdisciplinary pain management services throughout Australia, especially in regional and rural areas, worried Michael. Where services did exist, the 'waiting lists were diabolical'. At Royal North Shore Hospital, new patients languished on the waiting list for two years, while at Royal Adelaide Hospital, the average wait was four years. It was a similar situation across Australia.

For several days, Michael and Brydon talked through the findings and considered ways to improve access to pain services. They decided a national pain strategy was urgently needed. It would serve as a blueprint for best practice management of acute, chronic and cancer pain for all Australians. The pair agreed a necessary first step would be a consultation process with Australia's pain community to enable them to understand what was happening on the ground, particularly in regional and remote areas.

Armed with this information, they would assemble interdisciplinary working groups to draft a national strategy that would be presented to stakeholders for endorsement at a national pain summit. They were ambitious, wanting the strategy to convince health ministers around Australia of the importance of funding best practice treatment and management of acute, chronic and cancer pain as a health care priority.

Michael asked Brydon whether she would help manage the consultation and strategy development process and organise the summit, which they determined would be held at Parliament House in Canberra. 'Yes absolutely,' she said. And although she had no clear idea of what this would ultimately involve, she shared Michael's passion and commitment to address the problem and felt confident she could draw on her professional background to contribute to something significant.

Brydon herself had struggled with crippling pain for decades and knew how challenging it was to access the right services. She later told a journalist: 'I've suffered with arthritis since my twenties. I've had multiple joint replacements and spinal surgery. But I've learned to manage my chronic pain, where possible through diet, exercise and meditation, and tried to minimise my reliance on medications.'[137]

Agreeing the thrust of the strategy would be to set up a standardised interdisciplinary approach across the nation, Michael and Brydon set to work in mid-2009. They were determined to raise public awareness about pain—in particular, chronic pain—and the need for it to be treated differently from acute pain. It was a daunting task, but Michael believed it was possible 'if everyone involved in Australia's pain medicine community jumped on board'. He knew they would; they were all striving for the same thing—to improve pain management across the nation.

Michael approached the Australian Pain Society, the Australian and New Zealand College of Anaesthetists and Faculty of Pain Medicine, asking them 'to collaboratively lead the process'. They willingly signed on and agreed to provide some funding towards administrative costs. Aware of the urgent need to improve pain management, Dr Christine Bennett, CEO of MBF (now Bupa) was also keen to provide support and she committed MBF Foundation to help fund the project. Michael invited several leading pain medicine professionals to form a multidisciplinary steering committee and Brydon approached the Consumers Health Forum and Chronic Pain Australia for consumer representation.

The steering committee in turn formed three working groups and four reference groups to provide input on acute pain, cancer pain and palliative care, paediatric pain, and pain in older persons. Brydon also appointed an executive group to provide administrative support and following a tender process, selected the health journalist, Dr Norman Swan's, GSB Consulting and Communications to help manage the project. GSB's Rae Fry helped Brydon coordinate meetings, take minutes of every session and draft the strategy.

Steering committee members stipulated that the strategy must address the lack of pain medicine specialists in Australia. Pain medicine had been a specialist area of medical practice for five years by now, yet Australia had only two hundred qualified pain specialists. Most worked in public hospitals because Medicare and private health insurance funding was not available for interdisciplinary pain services—even though the Faculty of Pain Medicine had endorsed it as best practice. Services offered at private clinics were primarily pain management procedures such as nerve blocks, spinal cord implants and radio-frequency lesioning because they attracted Medicare and private medical insurance rebates. But few offered integrated psychology and physiotherapy services.'[138]

Simultaneously, Michael set out on a fact-finding tour to discover how other countries managed chronic pain. He wanted to know whether people with chronic pain could access interdisciplinary pain centres in other countries, how governments funded pain clinics, and whether other countries had national approaches to pain management. He travelled to the United States, the United Kingdom and several European countries.

During his travels, Michael continued negotiating with Royal North Shore Hospital's administrators about its redevelopment plans. When he returned, and after many months of sleepless nights spent worrying about the redevelopment, the hospital offered the pain centre a space in a small section of its main building. But Charles Brooker knew it would be inadequate for their needs. He felt it risked 'being whittled away' for other uses such as extra operating theatres and offices. Michael was keen to accept the allocation because he feared they might end up with nothing, but Brooker persuaded him to reject it. It was a risky move.[116]

Several more months of tense negotiations followed. Michael admits he 'got fired up at times' because he was determined to continue fighting until he had achieved an acceptable outcome. It was a monumentally stressful time in his life, but John Bonica had often told him: 'Get the facts right, son and never give up. Get the facts right and then persevere. Perseverance!' And this is exactly what Michael did. Dogged, he kept fighting, even when the going got so tough he lost all hope of saving the pain clinic. He recognises it can sometimes be challenging to pursue something you believe in but maintains that you must commit to staying the course despite the personal costs. 'When you're in a Cinderella position,' he said, 'it's easy for other people to stomp on you and be aggressive. It takes a lot of quiet determination. A lot of tenacity. It wouldn't have worked if I'd been outright aggressive, but I knew I had to hold my ground.'

Royal North Shore Hospital eventually offered the pain centre 1,500 square metres in its Douglas Building. The space was generous and would allow Michael and the team to design a state-of-the-art pain centre that better met the growing demand for pain management services. 'We only won in the twilight hours of the process,' Michael said. 'Once the hospital announced its decision, it wasn't all plain sailing because we had to move to a tiny space in the psychiatry department for two years while renovations proceeded on the Douglas Building.'

But the wait was worth it. When the new pain centre opened, pain research, education and the pain clinic occupied adjacent spaces, enabling pain patients to access an interdisciplinary team in a one-stop-shop.

During their decades of working with Michael, Kathleen Foley and Philip Siddall marvelled at how he handled challenging situations. Foley said Michael never pulled back when confronted by formidable opponents. His approach was, 'Well, what are our next steps? And the steps after that? How do we move this forward?'[21] Siddall agrees. He noticed Michael wasn't someone to lick his wounds and feel sorry for himself or give up. Instead, he pushed on a bit harder and thought of another way around the roadblock. 'Backtracking a couple of steps, he then did one of two things—either navigated around the obstacle, which was his preferred option, or retreated a couple of steps then tried again with a few more reserves on board.'[73]

Foley admired the way Michael was 'always in the trenches' doing research, treating patients and lobbying for improvements in pain management. 'He showed by his achievements how a person could be a high-level clinical scientist, a compassionate, skilled clinician and an advocate,' she said.[21]

15

NEW FRONTIERS

ONE of the techniques Michael watched as it evolved during the second half of the twentieth century was spinal cord stimulation. It first arrived in 1975 when the medical device company Medtronic started making the tiny electrodes required to transmit an electrical current. Michael said a major problem for researchers, even thirty years after devices first appeared, was that they didn't know how much spinal cord stimulation provided pain relief. 'Nobody had directly measured the properties of electrical signals along the spine,' he explains. 'In its early days spinal cord stimulation was rugged. It was a one-way system. You put in electrical pulses, but you didn't know what happened to them unless the patient said, "WOW, it's great, or it's terrible."'

Dr David Shearing at Flinders Medical Centre was one of Australia's first surgeons to implant a spinal cord stimulator. Michael was sceptical about the technology because he hadn't seen any scientific studies supporting its use. He often said as much to Shearing. 'As soon as you've got some scientific evidence, I'll take a much stronger interest in this.'

As research articles appeared in the pain literature about spinal stimulation, Michael started to implant spinal cord stimulators into his patients. Still, the technique was experimental, and he carefully explained its limitations to patients. Michael admits the device was often a 'last resort' for some patients with chronic pain.

To implant a stimulator, surgeons place two leads containing tiny electrodes into the space around the spinal cord. Then they connect the leads to an energy source similar to a pacemaker battery – positioned in the buttock or abdomen – to deliver a small amount of electrical current along the spinal cord. Pain specialists think the current reduces the constant state of heightened reactivity or wind-up in the central nervous system of people with chronic pain.

In an interview with *Australian Doctor*, Michael said in some patients, spinal stimulators can make a life-changing improvement. 'It can save them from going down the spiral of deterioration in mental and physical functioning that is so frequently seen in chronic pain.'[139] But the devices have major limitations and pain specialists don't know why they help some patients and not others. One issue is the stimulation often becomes too strong and can cause intense pain. 'When this happens,' Michael explains, 'most patients turn down the volume of stimulation to prevent these painful surges, reducing the amount of pain relief they receive.'

My own experience reflects both the benefits and risks of spinal stimulation. At one of my appointments with Michael, he suggested one option to ease my migraines was to implant a neurostimulator in my neck. 'It's a novel approach, and it's still experimental,' he warned. 'But I've tried it on a few of my patients who suffer from migraine, and it's helping them.' I was willing to take a risk because nothing else had worked. The first step was a trial run. Michael implanted the electrodes for one week, and miraculously, I had fewer migraines. Although it may have been a placebo effect, I went ahead with the surgery a month later to permanently implant electrodes. During the following weeks, I had fewer migraines than previously. I even had a few completely pain-free days. I felt as if Michael had given me my life back.

One year later, while washing my hair, I felt something sharp sticking out from the base of my skull. In a panic, I phoned the pain clinic, and the nurse told me to come in straightaway. Once there, I sat in the waiting room on a hard plastic chair trying to focus on what the morning television show presenter was saying. But I couldn't concentrate. My stomach was turning somersaults, and I was breathing too fast. After a while, Michael appeared, and he escorted me into his office.

After examining my neck, he said, 'I'm terribly sorry, but the end of the electrode has pierced the skin, and it's sticking out.' He took a swab and sent it to pathology, and I waited in the treatment room for the result.

A few hours later, Michael approached me. He wore a blue surgical gown and face mask. His face was ashen, and his shoulders stooped.

'I'm so sorry,' he said, 'but a golden staph infection is growing on the electrodes. I have to remove them. Otherwise, the infection won't clear.'

After the surgery, the migraines returned in full force, but three months later Michael implanted new electrodes. The second time around, they didn't relieve the pain as well, and I struggled with several migraines each week. Michael said it was possibly because of scar tissue blocking the electric current from doing its job. Still, overall I was better than before the first surgery. I worked full time, enjoyed weekly singing lessons and performed in the Sydney Philharmonia Massed Choir.

Two years later, I noticed a painful scab on the back of my neck. Michael swabbed it, discovering a superbug had infected the electrodes. The infection forced him to remove the electrodes again, plummeting me into a deep dark place. For several weeks after returning home from hospital, I carried around a portable intravenous device that delivered a continuous dose of the antibiotic Vancomycin. Community nurses visited me every day to maintain the infusion, making me feel like an invalid. During the following year, I lost a tremendous amount of weight, and once Michael re-implanted the electrodes, I still had migraines most days. Fortunately, I did the ADAPT program again, and it helped me better manage the pain.

Michael also implanted a neurostimulator into the neck of another of his patients, Symantha Liu.[86] Symantha had a decades-long history of migraine, and she too had 'tried everything'. At first, the device reduced her pain, but over time she found it progressively less helpful. She experienced a few issues, the major challenge being scar tissue covering the electrodes.

The scarring impeded the transmission of current, significantly reducing the device's stimulation capacity.[86]

Michael felt devastated by the complications Symantha, several other patients and I had experienced. He knew there was still 'a huge amount of room for improvement' and often phoned his colleagues, both in Australia and overseas, asking them about their experiences with spinal stimulation. Staying up late every night, he searched the latest research articles for clues.

In 2009, Dr John Parker, who had served as Chief Technology Officer at the hearing implant start-up company Cochlear, invited Michael to collaborate with him on developing a more sophisticated form of spinal stimulation than was available at the time. Parker was head of the Implant Systems Group at Australia's Information and Communications Technology Research Centre of Excellence (NICTA), which was later subsumed by CSIRO and subsequently spun out to become the medical device company, Saluda Medical. Parker longed to push the boundaries of technology he had worked with at Cochlear and believed one possibility was an advanced form of spinal cord stimulation for pain management. When he searched for the leading pain management expert in the region, Michael's name kept topping the list, so he decided to approach him. He called Michael's office three or four times and left messages, but Michael was busy and didn't return the calls. Determined to reach him, Parker contacted some of Michael's colleagues and asked them if they would speak with him about the idea. It worked and much to Parker's relief, Michael agreed to meet him.[140]

Michael and Parker first met in Royal North Shore Hospital's old brown building in September 2009. Peter Single, who had worked at Cochlear, was at the meeting, as was the pain research institute's, Dr Chris Vaughan.[113] Parker explained that he wanted to figure out how the spinal cord stimulators worked because no-one had yet done this.

'Neurostimulators send a current through the spinal cord,' Parker said, 'and doctors hope it produces pain relief, but they have no way of knowing what is going on in the spinal cord and whether it works. The only way they have of measuring the response is to ask the patient if their pain has improved.'[140]

The four men spent an hour talking about all the issues associated with bringing Parker's idea to fruition. Michael warned them it would be an arduous task. At the end of the meeting, he summed it up: 'We'll measure this thing no-one's ever measured before. We know it'll be difficult to measure, but if it works, we'll be able to see what the spinal stimulator is doing in the patient's body, and we may be able to see the underlying pathology of chronic pain. I don't think this will succeed, I think you're dreaming, but if it does, it will be vital, so I'll back you.' This response surprised Parker, who had not expected Michael to support the project.[140]

Meanwhile, Michael and Lesley Brydon continued to work on the *National Pain Strategy*. Michael and Brydon knew that to achieve a national approach they needed federal government support and endorsement for the strategy. They also hoped for government funding for development and a national rollout. But after several frustrating attempts, they couldn't secure a meeting with the Federal Health Minister, Nicola Roxon. Michael had spent decades lobbying politicians about the societal and personal costs of pain. Over the years, he had often shared research results that showed the impacts of interdisciplinary pain management—reduced suffering, disability payments, health care and pharmaceutical costs, and increased return to work after an injury. The pair hoped the economic lever of reducing disability payments and other health care costs through a national plan would be a catalyst for the federal government to embrace the strategy. But at this initial stage, they were unsuccessful.

While the MBF Foundation and several professional bodies had provided start-up funds to get the strategy process up and running, extra money was needed. Michael approached several pharmaceutical and biotechnology companies who agreed to collaborate, jointly contributing $250,000 by way of unencumbered educational grants. Providing these grants kept the contributions at arms-length to the strategy process.

The consultation process proceeded smoothly, and once the steering committee had completed its draft recommendations, Michael further developed and refined them. His drive to move the process along quickly astonished GSB's, Rae Fry, who assisted him with drafting. He often sent her handwritten notes late at night and on weekends, and he surprised her one Sunday morning when he phoned at seven o'clock to discuss the strategy.[141]

On 19 October 2009, four months after starting the project, the steering committee released the draft *National Pain Strategy* for public comment. Brydon issued a media release, sparking an avalanche of interview requests. In his interviews, Michael insisted the medical profession seriously mismanaged chronic pain.

'Currently in Australia and worldwide, it's fair to say pain management is shockingly inadequate,' he said. 'There is no other way to describe it.'

This situation has occurred due to inadequacies in knowledge, training, attitudes, practices, resources and structures. Pain is one of Australia's biggest health issues today, every bit as big as cancer, AIDS and coronary heart disease. Research has found that one in five Australians suffer from chronic pain, but less than ten percent are effectively treated.'[142]

Michael told journalists Australia urgently needed a public education campaign to promote understanding of chronic pain.

'There is a stigma around chronic pain,' he said. 'Some people with it are stigmatised as bludgers and copping out on their workmates. It's as cruel as that. There are lots of myths and myths are very, very hard to combat. We need to get the message out that chronic pain is a disease in its own right. I think today marks the beginning of an historic opportunity to address what we could describe as the largest undiscovered gap in health care, not just in this country but worldwide.'

In a radio interview the same day, Michael reiterated his message about the stigma associated with chronic pain. 'There are lots of myths about chronic pain—"You know, it's all in your head. You're just trying to get strong painkillers. You're just trying to get off work,"—and myths, of course, are very, very difficult to dispel.'

During this interview, Michael explained that pain that continues for more than three months produces physical, psychological and even environmental changes in a person and 'all of these add up to a disease entity just the same as any other disease'. His voice was resonant and measured. He added that recent brain-imaging technology had brought insights into how chronic pain can alter the brain. 'This imaging shows changes in the part of the brain that deals with sensation and motor function. What we've found is there are dramatic changes in the anatomy and even sometimes pathological changes that are associated with some of the nasty chronic pain conditions.' Citing spinal cord injury pain and phantom limb pain, he said: 'When one starts to see these changes in humans, it becomes a lot easier for people to believe that regardless of the condition that started the pain, additional pathology occurs in the nervous system that represents the disease of chronic pain.'[143]

Over the following weeks, the steering committee received forty-eight submissions from consumer and professional bodies, industry and individuals. Steering committee members reviewed 'every line of feedback', incorporating it into the draft strategy. They planned to debate it at the National Pain Summit a few weeks later. In the Foreword to the *National Pain Strategy*, Michael expressed his admiration of everyone involved in its creation: 'In more than forty-six years in health care, I have known no other health initiative to harness such a breadth and depth of experience on a single health problem. The most remarkable outcome has been the high level of agreement about what needs to happen in specific and practical terms.'[144]

A few months later, on Thursday 11 March 2010, the mood was electrifying in the Great Hall of Parliament House in Canberra as two hundred delegates including professionals working in pain management, mental health, rural health, and general practice, gathered to discuss the updated draft of the *National Pain Strategy*. Several patients and carers also took part. The summit aimed to reach a unified position.

The Federal Health Minister opened the event, which Dr Norman Swan, producer and presenter of the Radio National program, *The Health Report*, facilitated. Michael chaired the proceedings. He was excited although on edge because he realised the summit could be the beginning of a life-changing improvement in Australia's management of pain. It also represented the culmination of his four-decade quest to reduce suffering from pain.

In his opening address, Michael called on the federal government to appoint a task force to implement the *National Pain Strategy*. He also urged federal and state governments to back a community-led program to destigmatise chronic pain. The summit delegates, he said, had a responsibility to those with chronic pain, 'who are stigmatised, disbelieved, demoralised and grossly undertreated, resulting in complete destruction of quality of life, loss of employment and often impoverishment'.[145]

Describing how people with chronic pain face discrimination, he compared their management to people with other chronic diseases. 'Addressing this situation is a moral imperative,' he insisted, emphasising the last two words.[145]

Olympic swimming champion, Kieren Perkins, spoke about his former wife Symantha Liu's battle with chronic migraine. And the economist, Helen Owens, who prematurely left her senior government role because of poorly managed chronic pain, shared her story. Delegates heard from international pain experts, and following a day of intense discussion and debate, the strategy was unanimously supported.

The world's first *National Pain Strategy* provided a blueprint for the treatment of pain. It recommended an interdisciplinary approach to deliver best practice pain management. The delegates were euphoric. Many of them had volunteered their time to work on the many committees that developed the strategy, and they knew if the federal government implemented it across the nation, it would improve access to specialist pain management services for Australians who struggled with chronic pain. Later, the United States, Canada, England and several European countries would model their national pain strategies on Australia's.[144]

During the summit's lunch break, Michael did a radio interview on the national current affairs program, *The World Today*. He said the delegates were calling for governments and the medical profession to recognise chronic pain as a disease because it would improve treatment access. 'The moment chronic pain is recognised as a chronic disease and treated within the chronic disease category, patients will have more access to pain management services.'[146]

Michael told the interviewer it was a disgrace that eighty percent of people living with pain were untreated. 'For chronic pain, fewer than ten percent of those suffering from it can access effective treatment. Very simply, it's undertreated because it's not on the radar. I think this is a discrimination issue against patients with the disease of chronic pain compared to other chronic diseases.'[146]

In his interview, Michael noted Australia had an enormous opportunity to turn the situation around to enable people with pain to lead reasonably normal lives, get back to paid work and make a positive impact on the economy. 'It's time for the rubber to hit the road and for the federal government to set up an agency to implement the *National Pain Strategy*. The time is over for talking. This is a shameful situation. We need action—NOW!'

On the evening of the summit, Michael appeared on the Australian Broadcasting Corporation's flagship program *7.30 Report*. Despite a long day at the summit, he looked invigorated and much younger than his seventy-two years. His interview, 'Painful reality—patients let down,' was broadcast to a national prime-time audience. In a carefully modulated voice to maximise emphasis, he insisted that doctors and health professionals in Australia neglected people who suffered from pain.[147]

'Chronic pain isn't given the priority it deserves,' Michael told Kerry O'Brien, a prominent political journalist. 'The management of pain is shockingly inadequate. Myths abound in the general community, and I'm afraid to say this, across the medical and health care profession also, and a lot of people with chronic pain are subjected to not being believed, to implications they are trying to seek opioids, and even worse than that, that they're an opiate addict. And basically, they finish up receiving very unsatisfactory pain relief.'[147]

Michael explained to O'Brien that doctors and health professionals didn't understand the fundamental difference between acute pain and chronic pain and that the two conditions require different treatment approaches. 'For chronic pain, a team of health professionals must assess the patient to identify the various components of the problem and then a program that includes self-management, exercise and counselling needs to start. But this is just not happening, except in a very, very few pain centres. The important point to make is a wide range of treatments exist now for chronic and cancer pain and what we need is for patients to get access to these treatments. But they are being discriminated against inadvertently because we don't have the resources to provide that access. It should be a human right for people to have access to this treatment.'[147]

The *National Pain Strategy* provided Michael with a platform and he expertly used it to promote a message he had been trying to communicate for decades. Roger Goucke had taken part in the National Pain Summit, and its results impressed him. He assumed Michael had prearranged the outcome. 'He knew precisely what he wanted to come out of it.' Goucke admired how Michael 'lobbied, facilitated and organised, getting everyone together and ensuring they had their say. While his ideas were not universally accepted, most of them were.'[104]

Following the National Pain Summit, the neurologist, Leigh Atkinson, convinced the Queensland Health Minister to provide $40 million to improve pain services in Queensland. Atkinson believes this funding boost was a direct result of the summit. The Queensland government allocated enough funding to establish pain clinics at four of its leading hospitals.[148]

Associate Professor Paul Wrigley, a senior pain medicine specialist at Royal North Shore Hospital, had attended the National Pain Summit too and felt invigorated by it, believing it to be a step forward in improving pain management in Australia. In the lead-up to the summit, he had contacted an advocacy body within the New South Wales Department of Health – The Greater Metropolitan Clinical Task Force – urging it to embrace pain as a priority area of focus. A few weeks later, Paul Wrigley and Michael met with Dr Hunter Watt, the task force's head, proposing the state government develop a pain network to advise the health minister. Much to Michael's surprise and delight, Watt agreed. From that point, Wrigley and the pain medicine specialist, Dr Chris Hayes, established the New South Wales Pain Management Network, setting the wheels in motion for major reform.[149]

Summit delegates recommended the creation of a national advocacy body to help implement the *National Pain Strategy*. The Australian Pain

Society, ANZ College of Anaesthetists, Faculty of Pain Medicine and Pain Management Research Institute heeded the call, leading to the formation of Painaustralia.

Shortly after the National Pain Summit, IASP invited Michael to coordinate and chair its first International Pain Summit. Michael enthusiastically accepted, although he felt daunted by the prospect. Still, he believed the time was right to champion the concept of pain management as a human right, and he immediately set to work, assembling a steering committee to plan the summit's agenda. The steering committee included representatives of pain and palliative care organisations, human rights bodies from twelve countries, ethics consultants and individuals with publications on the topic. He discussed his idea with the steering committee, and its members agreed to pursue it. What followed was a lengthy process – via telephone and email – that involved representatives from sixty-two countries worldwide drafting, reviewing, editing and re-writing the *Declaration of Montreal*. Its simple message was: 'Access to pain management is a fundamental human right.'[150]

At the same time, Michael and John Parker collaborated on the neurostimulator project. From the start, they accepted the limitations of the currently available neurostimulators and recognised they must design a new device. They conducted initial experiments in Werribee, thirty-two kilometres south-west of Melbourne's CBD, using an off-the-shelf bio-amplifier and stimulator, where they recorded the first evoked response of a sheep spinal cord. Later, Michael and Parker conducted experiments on sheep in a sophisticated animal operating theatre in the basement of the Kolling Institute at Royal North Shore Hospital. Arriving early each day, they experimented with traditional spinal stimulator algorithms. They tested eight iterations of designs created by the NICTA team, testing the hardware on sheep, often working until late. Each iteration included features that took it closer to the goal of a tiny implantable device. Along the way, their studies confirmed the mechanism for spinal cord stimulation related to the Gate Control Theory proposed by Ronald Melzack and Patrick Wall back in 1965.

Confirming Melzack and Wall's revolutionary theory exhilarated Michael and gave him a much-needed energy boost. He was in his early 70s and found the early morning starts draining, especially when he had long conversations with his overseas colleagues about the *Declaration of Montreal* late into the previous night. But he believed the only way they would ever get any forward motion on spinal stimulation techniques was by getting concrete evidence. The sheep studies provided vital data, but Michael and Parker realised they needed to resolve several issues before permanently implanting the stimulators into patients. To prepare for this eventuality, Michael invited those staff who would one day operate on patients to join him in the animal operating theatre to help them gain experience testing the device using techniques similar to those they would use in humans.

Once Michael left the sheep laboratory each morning, he treated patients in the pain clinic and continued to navigate the draft *Declaration of Montreal* through the IASP hierarchy. But it hit a few roadblocks along the way because detractors argued that freedom from pain was not equal to access to clean water, education or freedom from slavery. Others argued it risked being grossly misinterpreted to imply everyone had the right to access opioids. These criticisms worried Michael. 'By the time I got it to the IASP council meeting, I sensed I'd have a tough fight getting it accepted,' he said. But to his immense relief, after a long and at times hostile meeting in Montreal later in the year, the IASP council approved the draft as a working document for the International Pain Summit.

In early September 2010, after the 13th World Congress on Pain in Montreal, IASP hosted its International Pain Summit. Over 260 association members from sixty-four countries, and representatives from professional and human rights organisations, assembled to debate the draft *Declaration of Montreal*. Michele recalls that Michael was nervous because he thought it would be an uphill battle to get agreement for the declaration. 'We thought it was just pushing too hard,' she said. 'It was definitely out there.'[5]

Despite his anxiety, Michael confidently delivered the opening remarks: 'Today we hope to address the tragedy of unrelieved pain.' But he worried the delegates wouldn't agree to accept the declaration because they thought it was too far-reaching.

The psychiatrist and pain medicine specialist, Professor Rollin Gallagher, served on the Summit Steering Committee, and he and Dr Philipp Lippe also served as the American delegates and speakers at the summit. Gallagher recalls the schedule was tight, with all sixty-four country representatives delivering a five-minute speech. 'The mood in the room was electrifying. Each delegate gave a short, impassioned presentation and we were running out of time because each participant gave such a powerful speech.' The consistency of delegates' messages astonished Gallagher, irrespective of whether they were from well-resourced countries such as Australia and America or developing nations. 'Everyone in the room was committed to the same thing—how to get good pain management into all countries. It was inspiring to be a part of it, and everybody shared the same feeling.'[151]

At the end of an intense day, a sense of euphoria filled the room when participants unanimously voted to accept the declaration. They had agreed to the right of all people to have access to pain management without discrimination; the right of people in pain to acknowledgment of their pain and to be informed about how it can be assessed and managed; and the right of all people with pain to have access to appropriate assessment and treatment of the pain by adequately trained health care professionals.[150]

'The delegates felt as if the pain medicine profession had come of age and had taken human rights on as a global challenge,' Gallagher said. 'It was exhilarating, and out of it came a determination to bring people from around the world together on pain education and training.' Gallagher believes the declaration empowered people interested in pain to persevere because they realised they had an international college of colleagues who supported what they were doing. 'We all hoped health professionals, human rights organisations, ethicists, governments and health care institutions would use the *Declaration of Montreal* as a resource to improve pain management.'[151]

However, a few opponents who have asked to remain anonymous report that peer pressure prompted them to vote in favour of the declaration. They question whether freedom from pain is the same as freedom from war, oppression or hunger, or immunising all children against crippling or deadly diseases. They ask whether pain is more important or less important than these other issues.

In an editorial published in the journal *Pain* after the summit, Michael and Mary Lynch, a professor of psychiatry, anaesthesiology and pharmacology in Canada wrote:

'The *Declaration of Montreal* is an important step in addressing inadequate pain management worldwide. Collaborative initiatives are now required among health professional and health policy organisations, human rights, legal and regulatory bodies with the overarching aim of 'Access to Pain Management as a Fundamental Human Right'. This aim should be addressed as a priority moral imperative. Success in achieving the aim will reflect the humanity of society.'[152]

One of the unexpected downsides of the *Declaration of Montreal* was that some people misinterpreted it to mean everyone deserved to be pain-free. 'In retrospect, some people consider this move may have contributed to the opioid crisis in the United States,' Rolf-Detlef Treede, a neuroscientist at the University of Heidelberg in Germany, said. 'This was not by design, but by misunderstanding. Our desire was to call attention to the need for a multimodal approach to the treatment of pain, not to say more access to opioids would solve the problem.'[153]

The opioid crisis is a grave public health issue in Western nations, particularly in America where 128 people died of an opioid overdose every day in 2018.[154] Like America, Australia experienced a large upswing in opioid use for chronic pain in the 2000s. Between 2010 and 2015, the number of prescriptions for opioids in Australia increased by twenty-four percent, largely driven by a sixty percent increase in oxycodone prescriptions.

Deaths due to opioid overdose also increased—from 3.8 to 6.6 deaths per 100,000 Australians between 2007 and 2016. The majority of these deaths were attributable to pharmaceutical opioids. In 2019, opioids accounted for just over three deaths each day. Most of these fatalities involved the use of pharmaceutical opioids, often in the presence of other substances.[155]

BREAKING THROUGH THE PAIN BARRIER

Roger Goucke disagrees with the assertion that the *Declaration of Montreal* contributed to overprescribing of opioids. He insists the statement means, 'We need to try our best to help people minimise their pain.' Goucke believes blaming the opioid crisis on the declaration takes out 'doctor judgement', that is, the fact that doctors will assess the patient and decide on the best approach to pain management.[104]

'Doctors are not just stooges for the opium industry,' Goucke asserts. 'You can't blame the opioid crisis on increasing interest in the effective and proper management of pain.'[104]

16

PAIN GETS A SEAT AT THE TABLE

ON 26 March 2011 the New South Wales Liberal Party won the state election, and Jillian Skinner became NSW's Health Minister. The previous year, when Skinner was the Shadow Health Minister, she had invited Michael to her Parliament House office. One of the issues they discussed involved Michael's worries about Royal North Shore Hospital's redevelopment plans and the furious competition for space. Michael felt downhearted at the time, but Skinner told him to 'hang in there' because if the Liberal Party won the state election she would give pain management the profile she believed it deserved.[156] Skinner had met Michael many years earlier and had visited the pain centre several times, so she was aware of the ADAPT program.[157] This was partly what motivated her to commit to a policy of developing a pain management plan as part of the Liberal Party's election platform.[156]

Around the same time, Painaustralia held its first board meeting in the Sydney offices of the law firm Corrs Chambers Westgarth. The board, chaired by the late James Strong AO, appointed Lesley Brydon as inaugural CEO. The West Australian Government donated $50,000 and the pharmaceutical companies again contributed, providing unencumbered educational grants, ensuring Painaustralia's voice and policy positions were independent. The advertising agency, Morris and Partners, worked with Brydon pro bono to develop the name and branding for the new organisation, and Corrs Chambers Westgarth developed the constitution, lodged a successful application for not-for-profit charity status and provided ongoing legal advice pro bono.[138]

Milton Cohen was the Faculty of Pain Medicine's representative on the inaugural board, and he recalls the mood of the first few meetings. 'Painaustralia was like a fledgling emerging from an egg and learning to fly,' Cohen said. 'But a tiny egg and a tiny fledgling.'[126]

Cohen admits it was tough trying to establish a not-for-profit organisation in the public health sphere. 'We were up against several high-profile charities such as Beyond Blue and the National Heart Foundation,' he said. 'Painaustralia's board members were trying to find their feet. They had two simultaneous tasks: to quickly gain a public profile and ultimately policymakers' and governments' attention. And they had to build a supporter base to attract donations and establish momentum.'[126]

Despite being a neophyte, Painaustralia's status as a leading voice in the pain world was recognised in mid-2011 when the European Parliament invited Michael and Lesley Brydon to Brussels to present the *National Pain Strategy*. Michael couldn't go because of commitments at the pain clinic but Brydon represented him. In an interview with *The Observer,* she said: 'Some of the most forward-thinking research on pain takes place in Australia. It is uncommon for non-Europeans to be invited to address the European Parliament, so it was great that we created something the rest of the world can take notice of.'[137]

Meanwhile, Jillian Skinner forged ahead with her plans. She changed the Greater Metropolitan Clinical Taskforce's name to the Agency for Clinical Innovation and instructed the agency to set up the New South Wales pain management task force. She asked Michael to join as an adviser, and appointed Professor Richard Chye, head of palliative care at Sydney's St Vincent's Hospital, as Chair. Skinner charged the task force with advising her on what she needed to do to implement a statewide pain management service.[156]

In May 2011, Skinner told journalists she had set up a task force to address issues raised at the National Pain Summit. 'It's vital for New South Wales to take the lead on delivering better pain management services,' she said. 'Severe and chronic pain has an enormous impact on sufferers, and on society as a whole. The costs, financial, emotional and mental, take their toll on everyone, which is why we must be better equipped to meet demand and try to reduce waiting times.'[158]

Jenni Johnson, the network manager for pain in the Agency for Clinical Innovation, played a lead role in the task force. She travelled to every pain clinic in New South Wales and interviewed the staff, asking them about their challenges and resourcing needs. Armed with this information, she briefed the task force, and they set to work.

'We used the *National Pain Strategy* like a skeleton,' Johnson said, 'applying its principles to the New South Wales plan and devising several recommendations that formed the plan's core. We wanted to ensure the New South Wales Government implemented interdisciplinary pain management across the state.'[159]

The task force members had a 'wish list'—they wanted a pain clinic in every health district across the state. They were determined to make existing pain management services sustainable because staffing was dwindling in some clinics. And they wanted to set up new services in regional and rural areas.

Johnson admired the way Michael worked behind the scenes with Jillian Skinner to manage the politics of the process. She noticed he never let the system daunt him, no matter how much resistance he faced.

'Michael just kept banging on the door with the same message that pain management was a human right, and everyone had a right to evidence-based treatment,' Johnson said. 'It was a powerful message. He took it to every meeting and started every discussion with it. Michael Cousins put pain management on the agenda in New South Wales and kept it there for many years, so it eventually became a government priority.'[159]

Simultaneously, Michael continued to pursue his political agenda at a national level. He believed it was critical to gain acceptance of chronic pain as a chronic disease in its own right, as distinct from a symptom of disease.

His goal was to use terminology that rightfully positioned pain in the minds of medical professionals, governments and the public to ensure it gained the prominence it needed to attract enough funding to improve its management. But when he and Lesley Brydon discussed it with senior health department officials they 'hit a brick wall', according to Michael. It didn't help that opinion among pain specialists was divided or that consumer advocates believed defining chronic pain as a disease may increase stigmatisation of patients. Brydon told Michael they had no hope of convincing the federal government of the veracity of the concept and that continuing to pursue it with them might alienate key health bureaucrats.

'It's one of the few times in my decade of working with Michael he looked dejected and as if he might give up,' Brydon said.[138]

Ultimately Michael agreed to move ahead with a more widely acceptable terminology for chronic pain as a chronic condition in its own right, rather than as a disease entity.

Despite its being a contested concept, Jillian Skinner supported the recognition of chronic pain as a disease. She led a move by the states, territories and the commonwealth to have the notion accepted and told Australia's Standing Committee on Health such a move would improve treatment and access to services for the one in five Australians who suffer from chronic pain in their lifetime. Recognising pain as a chronic disease, she insisted, would bring it into line with other diseases and validate it as a disease in its own right, not just a secondary disease or a symptom of something else. 'This recognition is essential so patients are identified earlier and can access the appropriate care they need,' she said.[160]

Concurrently with his political lobbying, Michael continued his early morning experiments on sheep. After months of fine-tuning, he and John Parker felt confident the latest version of the neurostimulator they were developing would help Michael's patients who suffered from chronic low back pain. Michael applied to Sydney University's human ethics committee and the hospital's ethics committee for permission to test the new device in five patients. Securing ethics approval was a long and complicated process, but both Sydney University and the hospital approved the project in 2012. Michael and Parker were finally ready to test the device.

Around this time, Michael rang the pain specialist, Marc Russo, and invited him to get involved with the research project. 'I'm not getting any younger,' Michael said. 'I need a young gun to push this on because these things can take a very long time to develop. We need someone with a busy pain medicine practice, a scientific vent and good ethics, and Marc, I would like you to clinically develop this with myself and John Parker.' At first, Russo had some misgivings about the project because of the difficulty of securing venture capital and getting a new medical device to market. But he said if an eminent professor asked you to do something, you don't refuse. 'I knew right there and then I was being given a rare lifetime opportunity,' he remarked. Still, as a busy pain medicine specialist he had little spare time and worried he would invest years in the project and the device might never 'see the light of day'. Russo asked Parker how long he thought it would take before the stimulator hit the market.[72]

'I've got absolutely no idea,' Parker admitted. 'Who knows how long it's going to take? It'll take as long as it takes. The important thing is to do it right, and then see where it leads. We'll work on this in the lab until it's as good as we possibly can do it. Then we'll be confident it'll help patients.'[72]

This response floored Russo, but he realised Parker was right. 'Michael and John Parker were not concerned about rushing something to market, or to put marketing spin on something half-baked. The pair had formed a powerful partnership in moving this project forward. Many, many people would have laughed at John Parker, and told him: "Go away. It's impossible, it can't be done." But Michael didn't do that, and as far as I was concerned, if Michael Cousins was backing it then I was happy to support it because if it worked it would revolutionise pain management.'[72]

The fourth patient Michael implanted with the device was an audiologist. Before the procedure, the NICTA team wheeled an enormous trolley into the operating theatre. Sitting on it were two computers and a bulky contraption sixty centimetres wide and sixty centimetres deep. They knew many more iterations of the design were necessary to shrink this

BREAKING THROUGH THE PAIN BARRIER

cumbersome hardware enough to implant into a patient, but they felt excited to have reached this stage in the project.

The audiologist walked into the operating theatre. Michael and Parker greeted her, and a nurse helped her onto the operating table. The anaesthetist sedated her, and a hushed silence fell over the operating theatre. Michael made a small incision in the audiologist's lower back and carefully inched the electrodes close to her spine. They were just to the left side of the midline.

Michael glanced at the anaesthetist. 'Half a millimetre of difference in position will produce a different area of stimulation. Now we need to see what the patient feels.'

The anaesthetist woke the patient.

'We're ready to do a trial stim now,' Michael told her. 'When I switch it on, we'll see live nerve responses. I'll move the stimulator to the spot that best blocks your pain.'

The audiologist nodded.

'Can you feel tingling?' Michael said.

'Yes,' the audiologist said.

'Where do you feel it?'

'In my left side.'

'Is it in your left back?'

'Yes.'

Later, when the team recorded the response of the audiologist's spinal cord to stimulation, a computer screen faced towards them.

'We can see the signals on the screen that show the device is stimulating the nerves in your spine,' Parker told her. 'As an audiologist you might find it interesting to see because similar technology is used in Cochlear implants.' He swivelled the screen 180 degrees, and the patient lifted her head from the pillow.

'I can't see anything,' she said. 'There's no signal.'

This response puzzled the team. When they returned the screen to its former position and as the patient returned her head to the pillow, the signal reappeared. They repeated the procedure several times but each time the patient lifted her head, the signal vanished.

'When I lift my head, the signal disappears and the tingling stops,' the audiologist said.

Parker said this response indicated that the size of the signal matched the strength of the sensation. By this time, the team knew that the variation in the strength of stimulation with posture and movement was a major problem in the industry. Medtronic had put an accelerometer in their implant to attempt to address it, but an accelerometer can't detect head position, so this solution was inadequate. Still, the team thought a feedback loop might solve the problem.

Over the following weeks the NICTA team added a feedback loop to the experimental stimulator set-up. Michael and Parker tested it on sheep. It worked![140]

One reason Michael was so determined to use a more sophisticated stimulator in his patients was the alarming spike in opioid use in patients with chronic pain. He wanted to find an alternative treatment for the millions of people worldwide with severe, unrelenting pain.

'All too often, people desperate for respite from their pain depend on a cocktail of opioids or other medications to get them through the day even though the drugs may not relieve their symptoms,' he said. 'We've known for decades that opioids rarely relieve chronic pain, but many doctors continue to prescribe them because they think it's their only option. They know pain clinics have long waiting lists, and they don't want their patients to suffer—so they prescribe one or more opioids and keep writing repeat prescriptions.'

People who suffer from chronic pain express the shame of being labelled an addict or drug seeker by medical professionals, family and society. And despite taking opioids, they often self-report a ten-out-of-ten pain score.

'For them, opioids are not helping to relieve their pain, but they may believe opioids are the only thing preventing even worse pain or a return to the pain levels before starting the medication,' Michael explains. 'Recent studies have shown the opposite is true—patients who took part in a carefully supervised opioid tapering program experienced reduced levels of chronic pain as they lowered their opioid consumption.'

Michael wants researchers to broadcast these results to educate patients and doctors—one of the principal reasons they avoid opioid tapering is fear of increasing the pain.[161] He hopes the government response to the opioid epidemic in Australia doesn't 'make the pendulum swing too far in the opposite direction', as it has in America. Rather than forcing people on long-term opioid therapy to suddenly stop taking the medication—to go 'cold turkey'—he believes a carefully tailored and monitored tapering plan is necessary to reduce the health risks associated with sudden cessation of painkillers. Also, he argues it is imperative that people with severe acute and cancer pain are able to access opioids.

'We need a coordinated effort to contain the opioid epidemic to maintain a balance between preserving access to opioids when clinically indicated and mitigating opioid-related harms,' he said.

Paul Hotz, a prominent Australian businessman and board director, started seeing Michael after struggling for over a decade with severe pain in his right knee due to a chronic staph infection. The pain and swelling were so bad his wife had to help him dress, and he walked using crutches and a walking stick. Paul had endured six rounds of surgery, and his doctors thought they might have to amputate his leg. They decided to try one more operation to determine whether amputation was their only option, and fortunately, it successfully removed the infection. But ten years of taking strong opiates had left Paul addicted to these drugs and, after the surgery, opioid addiction was his principal problem. Determined to kick the habit, he started therapy, and Michael supported him throughout this process.

'Michael acted as a conduit between what was happening to me physically and emotionally,' Paul said. 'He was an amazing support and helped me get off the opiates.'[162]

In mid-2012, Jillian Skinner asked Michael to host a press conference at the Pain Management Research Centre. He agreed, thinking the minister would use the occasion to promote the activities of the task force. Instead, at the event, Skinner announced the New South Wales Government had allocated $26 million over four years to fund the New South Wales *Pain Management Plan*.[163]

Michael was speechless. He hadn't realised the Minister's cabinet colleagues had agreed to fund the plan. Skinner told the assembled journalists the plan focused on integrating interdisciplinary pain management across all levels of the state's health system.

'I believe this is groundbreaking,' she said, 'because it's the first time that I'm aware of anywhere that there has been such a coordinated focus on pain management. It recognises this as an important chronic condition that has just been ignored.'[163]

Skinner explained the plan also included pain education, training and workforce development for health professionals, community-wide strategies to reduce the stigma of chronic pain, and better access to early intervention. When the minister announced extra funding for the Pain Management Research Institute, Michael's heart skipped a beat. The government had approved grants for the pain centre to boost its research, clinical services, the ADAPT program, and postgraduate education.[163]

'I couldn't believe what I was hearing,' Michael said. 'It felt like all my Christmases came at once.' Skinner confirmed Michael had no idea she would announce the $26 million in funding at the event. 'He almost burst into tears; he's such a humble and modest person.'[156]

The plan was a historic step forward in enabling a consistent interdisciplinary pain management approach across New South Wales.

Around the same time, Jane Cousins gave birth to a son. Michael and Michele were thrilled and flew to Milwaukee to stay with Jane, Charlie and baby, Henry. Michael loved being a grandfather. Jane said he was wonderful with babies and incredibly patient. 'When Henry cried, Dad walked around the house with him nestled against his chest, gently tapping his back.

He'd just walk and walk, doing laps and wearing holes in the carpet. He was definitely hands-on and loved being able to help me. He cherished that special time in our lives.'[68]

One year after Henry's birth, Parker and Michael were ready to trial their new 'closed-loop spinal stimulator' on patients. It was 2013, and although it had taken the pair over five years to reach this point, they felt confident their new technology would ultimately revolutionise twenty-first-century pain management.

17

CLOSING A CHAPTER

THE year 2014 was momentous for Michael. He turned seventy-five and desperately wanted to retire from Royal North Shore Hospital. But he had committed to remain in his role until the hospital had appointed his successor. The only stumbling block was that no-one seemed to want his job.[164] Still, his decades of relentless research and clinical care were recognised on Australia Day when he received one of the nation's highest honours—an Officer of the Order of Australia (AO)—for 'distinguished service to medicine through specialised tertiary curriculum development, as a researcher and advocate for reform and human rights in the field of pain, and as an author and mentor'.[165] Michael said he felt honoured by this recognition but insisted it truly belonged to everyone who had collaborated to advance pain medicine in Australia. When asked by journalists why he had devoted nearly five decades of his life to improving the treatment of pain, he told them his legendary story about the two burned boys: 'I was on duty one night at St George Hospital, and there was a message that two little kids were coming by ambulance. But they didn't come by ambulance—they came limping down the driveway. They had blackened faces, their hair was standing on end and they were screaming with pain.

They had burns to sixty percent of their bodies. They survived, and for the next few years, I looked after them. I suppose it was the first time I realised there were many conditions associated with severe pain that weren't well managed. Later, pain management was sewn into my subconscious when I trained in anaesthesia and intensive care and became interested in managing pain after surgery and trauma.'[164]

Several journalists asked Michael about his proudest achievement: 'Setting up the Faculty of Pain Medicine,' he told them. His colleagues agree. Leigh Atkinson asserts that setting up the faculty was a 'one-in-a-million skill' and it got people focused on chronic pain.[148] Marc Russo recalls that no-one believed Michael could get his idea off the ground, but he was formidable in overcoming the system inertia preventing the right thing being done. 'Michael got surgeons, physicians, psychiatrists, anaesthetists and rehab specialists into the room and told them of his plan to develop a Faculty of Pain Medicine, where each specialty would be represented. It says something about Michael's vision, wisdom, ethics and charisma that everyone knew they could trust him with this endeavour. The Faculty of Pain Medicine has a peerless reputation as an educational and accreditation body.'[72]

Dr Stephan Schug, a professor of anaesthesiology at the University of Western Australia, said that before the faculty existed, no-one saw pain as a priority. 'The faculty made pain visible to everyone and gave the pain medicine community power; it created political pressure for improvements in the system. Pain is something governments, insurance companies and the international community now talk about and the Faculty of Pain Medicine got the ball rolling,' Schug said.[166]

Roger Goucke believes the impacts of establishing the faculty are clear: 'Pain medicine specialists now have a seat at the table, and the federal government continually seeks inputs on policy from them, especially on issues surrounding the use of opioids.' Goucke admits the problem now is that the faculty is often snowed under with requests for input on many policies, which means it has to be agile to meet the government's short deadlines. 'It's now or never,' he said. 'The current Federal Health Minister, Greg Hunt, recognises the importance of pain, and he's consulting widely, which is a vital step forward. At least we're part of the conversation now. That would never have happened before Michael Cousins set up the Faculty of Pain Medicine. We can now influence health policy and Medicare item numbers.'[104]

Milton Cohen, who represented physicians on the original faculty board, was also the principal architect of the faculty's curriculum and training program. Cohen views Michael as a highly esteemed captain of the ship and is adamant that without his initiative, energy and political influence, the faculty wouldn't exist. 'Once Michael launched the ship, there were several lieutenants, and I count myself fortunate to have been one of them,' Cohen said. 'I think it's important to acknowledge the role of the captain.'[126] Russo agrees. 'To Michael, pain medicine was never about him. He was the leader who relentlessly drove forward with his vision. He worked long, insane hours until his late 70s. To him, advancing pain medicine was about wanting to reduce people's suffering. He wanted to leave our country in better shape.'[72]

The Faculty of Pain Medicine has accredited over thirty-seven pain clinics throughout Australia and New Zealand and over 365 pain medicine specialists currently practice in Australia. Fifteen of the practising specialist pain medicine physicians are GPs by background.[167] Given that pain is the number one reason people go to a GP and Australia has 36,000 GPs, Michael insists many more of them require training to gain specialist pain management skills.[168] He believes a possible deterrent is that the faculty's training program is full-time for two years. Participants work in an accredited interdisciplinary pain centre rather than remain in their general practice. The same barriers apply for medical specialists and surgeons.

Michael said these hurdles point to the need for greater availability of short courses across the nation to enable busy doctors to attend them. 'That's why we set up postgraduate programs and professional development at the pain centre,' he said. 'They're perfect for busy people because classes are on weekends or students can take part in the course online.' Still, despite some progress, Michael asserts our country needs many more pain specialists and specialist pain services to help the 3.24 million Australians suffering from chronic pain.

In February 2014, Royal North Shore Hospital renamed its pain centre 'The Michael J. Cousins Pain Management and Research Centre' to honour Michael's contribution to pain medicine over his 50-year career.[169] By that stage, he had helped thousands of patients, and published 236 scientific papers.[22] And several of his publications, including textbooks, were seminal in the anaesthesia and pain medicine literature.[44] According to Marc Russo, 'apart from the Gate Control Theory paper, Michael Cousins and Laurie Mather's 1984 review of the spinal route of analgesia is one of the most referenced papers in the history of analgesia.'[72]

In his speech at the renaming event, Michael once again acknowledged the herculean efforts of the pain centre's team in contributing to its success. He said it meant a lot to him to have the pain centre named after him.

'Thanks to all Pain Management Research Centre staff who helped me realise my vision,' he said. 'The Pain Management Research Centre represents more than anything else what I've been attempting to bring to fruition over the past twenty-three years in Sydney, and over the prior fifteen years in Adelaide.'[170]

When asked how he felt about the pain centre being named in his honour, Michael said: 'It's a mixed feeling. I'm pleased my efforts have been noticed. But there's a long way to go. Chronic pain is the next major illness in Australia after depression.'

In her speech at the renaming ceremony, Jillian Skinner acknowledged the contribution the pain centre had made to improving people's lives. She said its work had led to a new understanding of chronic pain as a disease in its own right.

'The Pain Management Research Centre revolutionised the way pain was managed and treated, bringing new hope and relief to many millions of people living with chronic pain all over the world.'[171]

Michael and John Parker hoped they would further revolutionise pain medicine with their closed-loop spinal stimulator. A decade earlier, Jaswir Grewel had completed the ADAPT program but several months down the track he realised the pain was once again taking over his life.

Over time, Jaswir relied on increasing doses of oral opioids and fentanyl patches to get through the day and felt as if he was 'falling into a dark hole'.

'I felt depressed and anxious,' he admitted. 'In a fit of desperation, my wife suggested I return to the pain clinic.'[83]

At Jaswir's appointment, Michael told him about the closed-loop stimulator.

'Would you like to try it?' Michael asked. 'You'd be the first person in the world to have it.'

Jaswir nodded. Michael explained to him that it might not work but Jaswir accepted this risk because if it helped him his life would 'irrevocably change for the better'.[83]

On 13 October 2015, Charles Brooker implanted Jaswir's device. Michael assisted with the procedure. Before the surgery, Jaswir said his pain was an eight out of ten, but it was a two out of ten after the surgery.[83][172]

'As soon as they turned it on the pain in my back disappeared,' Jaswir said. 'It gave me instant mental relief.'

In one of a series of media interviews about Jaswir's device, Charles Brooker told journalists: 'Spinal cord stimulators have been around for twenty to thirty years. They involve a wire sitting just outside the spinal cord, connected to a battery with a computer, just like a pacemaker. They send signals into the spinal cord, and so the person with pain feels tingling in the pain area, and that confuses the brain—they don't feel the pain, they just feel a pleasant tingling sensation.'

Brooker said unlike previous spinal cord stimulators, the closed-loop technology sent signals back from the body to help guide treatment. 'So that means the machine can adjust itself to produce whatever set level the patient wants. That's a big advance because previously, whenever people moved, or their heart was pulsating, various things would make the electrical signal waver up and down quite significantly. They would get shock sensations and not be able to live their lives effectively in many cases. This device is a big advance as it records the signal coming back out of the nervous system.'[172]

'It was a true Eureka moment in pain medicine!' Michael said. 'Conventional implants are blind to what's happening. They pump out a signal. They can talk, but they can't listen. In comparison, the closed-loop device enables a two-way conversation. It's the first device where the stimulus adjusts in response to feedback from the patient's nervous system, optimising the level of pain relief. So by listening, the device regulates the amount of stimulus to match the level of pain, giving a dose of pain relief tailored to the patient's needs at the time.'

Michael said another advantage of the system was that patients didn't experience unpleasant sensations when the device provided too much stimulation. He recalls one of his patients who had a traditional spinal cord stimulator used to grab a nearby wall or bookshelf to brace himself whenever he coughed. 'He did this because he received a massive overstimulation from a percussion wave travelling through the spinal cord—the spinal cord whipped,' Michael said. 'His experience was like having a little electric shock. In some people, it knocked them off their feet because it hurt so much. The patient ended up turning down the level of stimulation, reducing his pain relief, but preventing the unwanted overstimulation.'

Repeated studies in Australia and overseas revealed that overstimulation, shocks and thumping don't occur with a closed-loop system, enabling patients to maintain a constant stream of stimulation and pain relief, even when they cough.[173] [174] Michael recalls one patient's response when they turned on the closed-loop stimulator.

'Oh yeah, I feel a difference,' the patient said, beaming. 'At first, I have a sort of tingling, and then the pain disappears. There's none of the thumping and buzzing going on. It just takes the pain away.'

Michael explained to the patient the thumping sensation she had noticed with her old stimulator was her heartbeat. 'The spinal cord contracts and swells with every heartbeat and this can increase the stimulation to a painful level,' Michael told her. 'In some patients, the older-style stimulators effectively turned off with every heartbeat. This meant it switched on, off, on, off, on, off all the time. The pins and needles and the thumping were the motion the spinal cord superimposed on the sensory input.'

Following Jaswir's surgery, Michael and Allan Molloy supported him while he slowly tapered his opioid use. Now he is thrilled to be entirely drug-free.

'The stimulator has taken over my pain control,' Jaswir said. 'It's doing all the work of the opiates and other pain medications I took. My spinal cord stimulator is the best thing that ever happened to me.'[83]

Michael feels ecstatic about the closed-loop stimulator. He hadn't expected it to provide such effective pain relief. He feels he's come full circle since the evening he wrote his application for a postgraduate fellowship to study in Montreal with Philip Bromage. In his application, he had proposed placing electrodes into the epidural space to provide pain relief.

'At the time, I didn't think it would take me nearly half a century to reach this point, but I'm glad I persisted,' he said. 'The closed-loop stimulator is a powerful example of the close integration of research and clinical care, a practice John Bonica tirelessly advocated. I always encouraged this integration throughout my career, but it was an uphill battle to get the scientists and the clinicians to collaborate. I'm so grateful John Parker as a scientist chose me to partner with him. Working with him is the best experience I've had in my career. It takes me back to my collaborations with Charlie Wright at McGill and Richard Mazze at Stanford'.

In 2015, Michael was delighted when his son Chris became a father to twins—Richard and Mila. After his twin's birth, Chris took a year off work to look after them. Michael wishes he too had taken a break to spend time with Jane and Chris when they were born. He regrets being so busy with work when his children were young.

The year after Chris' twins were born, Michael retired from Royal North Shore Hospital. He was bone-tired and had wanted to retire years earlier, but the hospital 'took forever' to replace him. 'I felt shattered with exhaustion,' he said, 'but I didn't want to leave the pain centre in the lurch and committed to stay put until my replacement started. I shouldn't have stayed so long because it irreversibly impacted my health—for the worse.

On the other hand, I didn't want the pain centre to lose momentum if I departed before someone else took over its leadership.'

Michael was relieved when Dr Paul Glare, a prominent palliative care physician, agreed to lead the pain centre. The two pain specialists had crossed paths several times during the 1990s and 2000s and Glare had taught the cancer modules of Sydney University's Master of Pain Management program. He was head of pain and palliative care at Memorial Sloan Kettering Cancer Center in Manhattan and was sitting in his office in New York one day when he read the advertisement for Michael's role. The next day Michael telephoned him in New York, encouraging him to apply. Every morning for the following week, Michael called Glare, urging him to consider the position. In the end Glare relented. He flew to Sydney for an interview and the hospital offered him the role a couple of months later.[90]

On 19 May 2016, Michael's last day at Royal North Shore Hospital, the pain centre hosted a Festschrift presentation to celebrate his career. Jillian Skinner, pain centre colleagues, and leading pain medicine experts from Australia and worldwide, paid tribute to him during the event.

In his speech, Charles Brooker said Michael's vision for the future is unique. 'First, he has an idea,' Brooker said. 'Next one hears the idea mentioned and seemingly overnight, it just happens.' Brooker listed the many textbooks Michael wrote or edited, the three hundred journal articles, the NHMRC Centre of Excellence, ADAPT, the master's courses, the recognition of pain medicine as a specialty, the Faculty of Pain Medicine, the National Pain Summit, the *National Pain Strategy* and the New South Wales *Pain Management Plan*. Brooker said it all seemed effortless, but all these things dramatically impacted the availability of care for patients. Brooker also mentioned how he had appreciated the chance to learn from Michael how to survive hostile hospital meetings on the topic of funding—'a dark art!'[175]

The event concluded with Michael receiving a *Festschrift*—a book chronicling his achievements.[176] As he accepted it, he said: 'Being exposed to people like John Bonica stimulated in me a great sense of responsibility to the field of pain medicine and to the patients I treated. I'm always trying to decide whether I'm meeting my obligations to the field of pain medicine and my patients. It's immensely satisfying to be able to treat patients whom no-one else could previously help—it's not only satisfying, it's exhilarating! I think it's a field that's enormously demanding. It's incredibly debilitating sometimes to deal day after day with patients for whom sometimes you can do nothing. It can sometimes grind you down. But the potential rewards are very great, and I think it's a wonderful area of medicine to practice, no doubt about it.'[177]

After Michael retired, he continued his research on the closed-loop spinal stimulator with John Parker. The latest generation device continuously and instantaneously adjusts the level of spinal cord stimulation, preventing both under stimulation and overstimulation.[178] At Royal North Shore Hospital, Dr Charles Brooker, Dr Nathan Taylor, Dr Martine O'Neil and Dr Rebecca Martin have implanted the device into several patients who have experienced significant pain relief.[116] Michael is thrilled that patients at the Pain Management Research Centre can access the closed-loop system and benefit from each new iteration of this transformational treatment option.

Twelve months after he retired, Michael, John Parker and an extensive research team published a pivotal study known as the *Avalon Study* about the progress of thirty-six patients with chronic back and leg pain whom they implanted with the new neurostimulators.[179] Most patients still experienced substantial pain relief eighteen months after their surgery. In a later study of different patients, seventy percent of them reported eighty percent improvement in pain relief eighteen months after the device was implanted.[173]

In 2020 the research team published another study of outcomes. The team assessed ratings of pain, quality of life, function, sleep and medication use in fifty patients with lower back and leg pain before implanting the device, then at regular intervals following surgery. Most patients experienced over eighty percent pain relief one year after surgery.[174]

Michael feels hopeful, given the improvements in patients' pain scores have been steady, which he previously never witnessed with traditional stimulators. Charles Brooker believes the study results are encouraging.

They suggest pain relief continues to improve over time, which rarely happens with the older systems.

'The closed-loop stimulator is a significant advancement to the field of pain management,' Brooker said.[116]

According to Marc Russo, Michael's early neuromodulation work commenced in 1979 around spinal and epidural delivery of opioids for pain relief. This research, a long-term collaboration with Laurie Mather, was one of the founding pillars of knowledge in this area. 'For some men this would warrant resting on their laurels, but this was followed with a prodigious output on spinal cord injury pain management,' Russo said. 'Michael's interest in neuromodulation never wavered and he added spinal cord stimulation to his clinic's armamentarium in the 1990s. In 2009, he began a collaboration with an engineer with wild ideas on measuring action potentials in the spine and his scientific foundational work and intellectual support has helped the imminent birth of a home grown commercially available spinal cord stimulator system.'[72]

Many of the impacts of Michael's decades of dedicated research, clinical care, teaching and advocacy are now bearing fruit. Kathleen Foley said Michael played a pivotal role in advancing the international field of pain medicine, 'setting a high bar for pain research, pain education, training in pain and for advancing the field globally'. She respected the way he relentlessly pursued novel approaches for treating pain and continuously drove the science of pain medicine with his discoveries by working 'in the trenches doing research'. Foley recalls that during Michael's term as IASP President his advocacy skills set him apart. She admired his eloquence, powers of persuasion and calm demeanour, even in the toughest situations. 'Whenever IASP lobbied governments and influential organisations and required leadership, Michael 'was the person IASP wanted out front'.

Michael's advocacy skills have also borne fruit in Australia and he had a knack for eliciting enthusiasm from others for the cause. One of the key supporters for his work was influential Managing Director of Corrs Chambers Westgarth, Robert Regan, who chaired Painaustralia's board for eight years. Regan brought a commitment to getting pain management on the national agenda and was able to govern the organisation from its early inception to achieve Michael's vision of becoming a strong national peak body for the sector that it is today.

Since its inception, Painaustralia's lobbying has gained increasing traction, and the federal government now recognises the need to improve pain management. In 2017 when Lesley Brydon retired, Michael urged former Consumers Health Forum chief, Carol Bennett, to apply for the CEO position.[180] She eventually agreed and the Painaustralia board appointed her.

The following year the federal government provided seed funding to enable Painaustralia to create a *National Strategic Action Plan for Pain Management* based on the *National Pain Strategy*.[181] Twelve months later, the Federal Health Minister, Greg Hunt, committed $6.8 million over four years to improve pain management across Australia.[182] Painaustralia received $1 million to educate people living with pain, and the organisation used some of the funds to build an interactive website. The federal government also allocated funding for rural health outreach programs and to upskill general practitioners. Michael said this funding is a good start, but it is a 'drop in the ocean' and governments need to invest much more to provide pain management services across the nation.

In mid-2019, Carol Bennett launched the *National Strategic Action Plan for Pain Management,* which sets out the key priority actions to improve access to pain management across Australia to ensure everyone in pain can benefit. In 2021, the plan received full endorsement from all Australian health ministers. 'Gaining support from all state health ministers was vital for implementing a consistent approach to pain management, especially in regional, rural and remote areas where specialist pain management services and community support are in short supply,' Bennett said.[183] 'This means we'll have a truly national approach to pain management. It'll also mean we'll need to continue to advocate for resourcing of the plan to ensure it can achieve its full potential.'

In Australia, New South Wales was the frontrunner in introducing a statewide pain plan, but other states soon followed. Recent funding of pain programs by state governments has reduced the time people with chronic pain wait to see a pain specialist. However, many people report languishing on a waiting list for twelve months or more, which points to the need for more accessible pain management services.[184]

Many online resources are now available for people who cannot access a public pain clinic or an affordable pain specialist. One example is the Agency for Clinical Innovation Pain Management Network run by the New South Wales Government that helps people better manage their pain.[185]

It also includes resources to educate general practitioners. Recently, support groups for people with chronic pain have sprung up around the country—the Australian Pain Management Association[186] and Painaustralia list contact details for these groups' organisers on their websites.[187] Also, Chronic Pain Australia provides educational resources on its website and a forum to enable people living with pain to support each other.[188]

Michael's advocacy for access to pain management to be a human right is also gaining currency. The World Medical Association endorsed the declaration's principles in 2011, resulting in the International Federation of Health and Human Rights Organisations making it one of its two top priorities. The World Health Organization now supports the concept, raising its emphasis on pain management in its global health programs.[189] The European Pain Federation's *Societal Impact of Pain* platform,[190] the United States Institute of Medicine's *Relieving Pain in America* report[191] and the US *National Pain Strategy*[192] also referenced the declaration. In a 2019 speech to the International Neuromodulation Society, Marc Russo said Michael's advocacy on human rights 'has led to generational, institutional, and governmental change in the way human beings are treated on this planet whether that be survivors of torture or dementia patients or Third World access to analgesics. For this alone, Michael, we applaud you'.[22]

A 2020 review of the *Declaration of Montreal* concluded that it brought the concept to the attention of politicians, policymakers and health professionals globally and has helped shape advocacy and policy regarding pain management. The review stated: '*The Declaration of Montreal* highlighted the inadequacies of access to pain management resulting from factors like the stigma of chronic pain with or without a diagnosis, a dearth of health care education regarding the mechanisms and management of pain, and a lack of national policies concerning pain as a health issue in its own right.'[153]

The concept of chronic pain as a disease is still debated in pain circles today, but despite a lack of consensus about it, the notion underpins the National Pain Strategies of Australia and the USA, and the New South Wales *Pain Management Plan*.[4] [192] [193] It was also a vital principle of the National Academy of Sciences Institute of Medicine report to the US Congress: *Relieving Pain in America, a Blueprint for Transforming Prevention, Care, Education and Research*.[194] In 2018 the Australian Government included pain management in its Medicare review, recognising chronic pain as a chronic disease.[136] [38]

The International Association for the Study of Pain recently brought some clarity to the debate when it published ten papers in its journal *Pain* outlining an updated and more highly nuanced classification system for chronic pain.[195] In May 2019, the World Health Organization adopted a new edition of its *International Classification of Diseases (ICD-11)* that systematically represents chronic pain diagnoses.[196] *ICD-11* is the first version of the *ICD* to include chronic pain, and it based the classification on the recommendations of an IASP task force. IASP welcomed the inclusion of chronic pain in *ICD-11*, saying it is one way to 'ensure chronic pain receives greater attention as a global health priority. It is the hope of the [IASP] task force that the inclusion of the chronic pain conditions in the *ICD-11* will further the recognition of chronic pain as a health problem in its own right and contribute to improved access to adequate pain treatment for persons with chronic pain worldwide.'[195]

Marc Russo admires Michael's vision and the way he played the long game. Even if a problem seemed insurmountable, Michael recognised that by relentlessly 'chipping away, nudging and pushing' he would crack it a couple of years later. Russo believes people like Michael come along 'very, very rarely,' and sometimes they are fully appreciated inside their working lifetime, but often the true scale of what they achieved is only understood with the passage of time—mostly years or decades later. 'Michael is one such person who was recognised for what he achieved within his working lifetime, and he continues to receive awards, and accolades beyond that,' Russo said.[72]

'Michael Cousins was a force of nature in what he was able to achieve, and what he achieved was to convince people of his vision and corral them into working alongside him to achieve that vision,' Russo explains. 'As well as doing that with his anaesthesia and pain medicine colleagues, he did it across hospital units, hospitals, state boundaries and even national borders. He was able to convince hospital bureaucrats to release money, and support a very unattractive, unsexy area of medicine. He was very well connected politically and had the ear of prime ministers at times. He convinced politicians to pour money into an electorally dead area of medicine. He didn't achieve all this through dictatorship or bluntness in personality. He achieved it by appealing to people's good nature and explaining to them how much more could be achieved—indicating to them that the status quo wasn't acceptable, and the status quo was only a fraction of where things could go.' Russo said he learned a lot from Michael and attended many of his lectures. But he wishes Michael had given a lecture on how to access politicians and motivate them to do the right thing. 'I wish I'd learned some of his political and negotiating skills because they were very effective.'[72]

Michael's pursuit of his vision to reduce suffering by improving pain treatment drove his decades of pain research, clinical care, education and advocacy. It gave him the indefatigable energy he required to move mountains in the face of funding shortfalls, the efforts of opponents, complacency and systemic resistance to change. Michael, Michele and their children made untold sacrifices along the way, and Michael faced seemingly insurmountable challenges at times. He also experienced his share of disappointments, but he never gave up, persevering until he achieved his vision.

Like many pioneers, Michael always focused on the end game rather than the small steps along the way. Notably, he depended on his talented colleagues to complete the many projects he had started. Still, maybe an unrelenting focus on the big picture and crusade-like approach is what it takes to bring about a fundamental reform of treatment protocols, national health policies, institutions and attitudes. While there is still a long way to go to provide access to pain management services for everyone who needs it, Michael's driving vision indisputably advanced pain medicine in Australia and around the world. It has given hope of a better life to countless people worldwide.

In conclusion, it is probably best to let Michael's patients articulate his legacy because his quest was to reduce their suffering by improving pain treatment. Michael's patients speak of his tireless devotion to helping them better manage their pain. They accepted his inability to cure chronic pain, but they all say he gave them hope. Patient after patient noticed and appreciated Michael's habit of worrying about them until he landed on a solution to reduce their pain and suffering. And they felt he truly listened to them, something they had rarely experienced during their years of struggling with pain. Paul Hotz maintains Michael gave him the power to cope with life[162] and Michael's patient, Robyn, believes his kindness and care saved her sanity.[82] They both say he is charming and compassionate, but not judgemental or dismissive. 'He listens, takes us seriously and goes over and above to help us,' Robyn added.[82]

Symantha Liu's most vivid memory of Michael involves a hospital ward and a tuxedo. She had been suffering with a cluster migraine for several days when the pain became unbearable. Michael admitted her to Royal North Shore Hospital for care and observation, and at one point, the pain was so bad she begged the nursing staff to 'just knock me out'. Symantha was continually vomiting, dehydrated and sobbing from the pain.

'The migraine was impacting my vision, and I had never felt so vulnerable,' she said. 'I thought death would be better.'

A little while later, Symantha felt a gentle hand on her shoulder and heard a soft voice say: 'Sam, it's me, Michael.'

Through her tear-stained eyes and blotchy vision, she struggled to make him out. Slowly a man wearing a dashing dinner jacket and with dapper silver hair came into view. He was almost luminous, and in her state one thought came to mind.

'Am I dead, Michael? Is it really you?'

Michael chuckled quietly and told Symantha he was still beside her and not to worry. She asked him why the hospital had disturbed him if he had somewhere important to be.

'Whenever I feel one of my patients has reached a migraine crisis, I can only feel better if I lay eyes on them for my own peace of mind,' he said.

Symantha says this is the measure of the man. 'For me, forever, a saint on earth.'[86]

EPILOGUE

FOLLOWING his retirement, Michael continued his research with John Parker and treated patients at the pain clinic at North Shore Private Hospital. While he missed his colleagues, many of whom were lifelong friends, he was relieved he never again had to sit in a meeting with a hospital administrator. According to Marc Russo, Michael's 'seriously honed negotiating skills' with bureaucrats were legendary and he, like his colleagues, had often seen Michael 'gently guide administrators into decisions they hadn't realised they needed to make'. Russo recalls one way Michael kept his cool during long evening meetings was to pour a nip of Johnny Walker Black Label Whisky into a glass and slowly sip it. 'It helped him endure those whose verbiage exceeded their intellect.'[22] With those frustrating meetings a distant memory, Michael embraced leisure time for the first time in his adult life. Catching gigantic waves on his surf ski at Palm Beach filled many days, as did playing golf with Michele and spending time with his grandchildren. He also relished the chance to read novels and biographies and watch the Wallabies play rugby.

At the beginning of 2018 Michael was very ill with pneumonia. He took several months to recover and lost a considerable amount of weight. He retired from private practice in June and later in the year his neurologist told him he had Parkinson's Disease. It was a devastating blow, and Michael regretted that he hadn't retired earlier when he was in robust health. While his habit of navigating around roadblocks had served him well during his career, Parkinson's was less amenable to negotiation and charm. It was a formidable obstacle, but in true Michael Cousins style, he tenaciously applies himself to living the best life he can despite his illness. He and Michele still try to go to concerts and play golf, and they walk and swim at Palm Beach. Michael has paddled his beloved surf ski on Pittwater a few times with help from his sons and friends, and he spends as much time as possible enjoying the company of Michele, his children, grandchildren, extended family and friends.

Michael's two great loves are his family and medicine, and he is happiest when his family is together at his home. Throughout his career, he loved the thrill of a new medical discovery. But most of all, he loved helping people better manage their pain. He longed for them to resume their pre-injury activity levels and be able to live a good life.

These days Michael likes to catch up by phone with his pain medicine colleagues in Australia and across the globe so as to keep in touch with the latest developments in the pain world. He is looking forward to a future where Australia's *National Pain Strategy* helps to reduce suffering from pain, and where no-one need endure the horrific pain suffered by the two burned boys he treated at St George Hospital over fifty years ago.

AFTERWORD

I first met Michael Cousins when he was spending every spare minute pulling together the National Pain Summit in 2010. Michael understood the politics of getting as many key peak bodies engaged in championing the need for pain to be placed on the national agenda. It has never been done before. I was the CEO of the Consumers Health Forum of Australia and his energy and enthusiasm convinced me this was an event we needed to be part of. Michael convinced all of us the summit could change the way the health system treated people experiencing chronic pain. This was clearly a life-long passion and Michael went to great lengths to co-opt all the people he believed could make a difference in this area.

It was no mean feat to pull together 150 key players for a meeting in Canberra, all fully sponsored and attracting important politicians and policy makers who could drive the national health agenda. The recommendations of the summit led to the development of Australia's first national pain strategy which provided a very important platform for recognition of pain and evidence-based approaches to its treatment.

Seven years later, I had the great fortune of hearing from Michael again, this time to discuss the national peak body he had founded and its search for a new CEO to replace founding CEO Lesley Brydon. While the organisation had made great strides forward, especially with state governments, the need to enlist the support of the federal government more firmly in a national approach remained. At first, I was a little reluctant, but it can be hard to say no to Michael. He did not let go. Several weeks and numerous conversations later, I was convinced that Painaustralia had the potential to deliver real change in an area of health that had been sadly neglected over many years despite its impact on individuals, families, workplaces and communities. I became the Painaustralia CEO.

Four years on, the *National Strategic Action Plan for Pain Management* (the blueprint for action to achieve the objectives outlined in the *National Pain Strategy*) has been endorsed by all states and territories and the federal government is exploring the possibilities for launching the Plan. This will be a world first practical and national approach to pain management.

Michael has been the change maker that people living with chronic pain in Australia (and indeed around the world) needed. His legacy is profound.

Most people who experience the agony that is chronic pain will not know of Michael. Neither will their families, their work colleagues, or their communities. But because of Michael, pain is now a national health issue with a clear plan of action and an army of people ready to go to work.

For me, Michael is one of those rare lighthouse figures, showing us the way, and in so doing demonstrating what a remarkable, dedicated man driven by a passion and persistence can achieve.

Carol Bennett, *CEO, Painaustralia*

painaustralia

NOTES

1 LEARNING ABOUT PAIN

i   Regional anaesthesia is the use of local anaesthetics to block sensations of pain from a large area of the body, such as an arm or leg or the abdomen.

2 MONTREAL

ii   TENS is transcutaneous nerve stimulation. A TENS machine passes electricity across the skin to stimulate nerves and relieve pain.

6 THE RACE TO ADVANCE EPIDURAL PAIN RELIEF

iii   The dura is the outermost fibrous membrane covering the spinal cord.

14 THE 2000s

iv   The Great Schism of 1054 marked the split of Christianity and established the separation between the Orthodox Churches in the East and the Roman Catholic Church in the West.

ACKNOWLEDGEMENTS

MICHAEL and Michele Cousins generously opened their home to me every Wednesday afternoon for months on end until COVID-19 hit, and we convened using Facetime. Our weekly interviews felt like we were reliving the memoir *Tuesdays with Morrie* by Mitch Albom. Michael patiently answered my hundreds of questions and provided me with access to his private archives and photo albums. He also opened doors to the pain world, introducing me to people across the globe who, like him, had shaped pain management as we know it today. My heartfelt thanks, Michael and Michele. I know it was difficult to have someone probing into your private life, but you were unendingly open and gracious, and I deeply appreciate it.

I'm eternally grateful to the dozens of family members, colleagues, patients and friends I interviewed, sometimes multiple times—Dan Carr, Philip Siddall, Charles Brooker, Allan Molloy, Carol Bennett, Jane Kuehn (nee Cousins), Geoff Cousins, John Parker, Kathleen Foley, Milton Cohen, Jillian Skinner and Paul Glare. And thanks too to Michael's patients who trusted me with their intensely personal stories.

Thank you to everyone who reviewed, fact checked and commented on draft after draft of the manuscript—Fiona Giles, Susan Thomas, Judith Godden, John Loeser, Marc Russo, Laurie Mather, Lesley Brydon, Carol Sklenicka and my ever-supportive and loving husband Ian Davies.

Breaking through the pain barrier was funded by a grant from the Pain Management Research Institute at Royal North Shore Hospital. I would like to thank Brian Davidson and the Pain Foundation Board for providing this funding, without which the book wouldn't exist.

And an enormous thank you to Carolyn Martinez from Hawkeye Publishing for believing in me and my manuscript. I deeply appreciate your enthusiasm, sensitive editing and support.

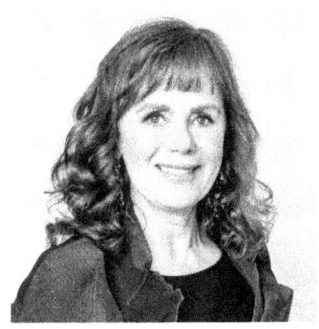

ABOUT THE AUTHOR

BIOGRAPHER Gabriella Kelly-Davies has been writing stories ever since she mastered the alphabet—now that passion has seen her win three writing prizes. Gabriella has studied life writing at Oxford University, Sydney University and the Australian National University and she is a doctoral student in biography. She is the founder of Share your life story and has written over thirty self-published memoirs, life stories and family histories for her clients. Gabriella is President of Life Stories Australia Association and believes the art of biographical storytelling is a particular writing genre—it's not fiction, but it requires the weaving of someone's life story into a form that compels readers to keep turning the pages to find out what happens next.

'I'm passionate about storytelling and helping people share their story. Life writing is a powerful way of communicating what you stand for, the lessons you've learned in life, the exciting journeys you've embarked upon and the knowledge you've gained through life's ups and downs. From an early age, my dad took me to the local library every week to borrow biographies of musicians, writers, artists and political leaders. I love getting to know fascinating and inspiring people through their life stories—what it's like to be them living their life; their motivations, experiences, relationships, passions and struggles. It's a great privilege to read someone's biography and an even greater privilege to write them.'

BIBLIOGRAPHY

1. Hilton J. *Rest and Pain.* 6th ed. Walls EW PE, Atkins HJB., editor. Philadelphia: J. B. Lippincott Co; 1950.
2. Cousins MJ. *Anaesthesia Stories.* Professor Michael Cousins. [Interviewed by: Scott, D.] Faculty of Pain Medicine, 2017.
3. Bonica JJ. *The Management of Pain* Philadelphia: Lea & Febiger; 1953.
4. National Pain Summit Initiative. *National Pain Strategy.* Sydney; March 2010.
5. Cousins Michele. Personal interview. 22 May 2020 [Interviewed by: Kelly-Davies G].
6. Cousins MJ, Wright CJ. Graft, muscles and skin blood flow after epidural block in vascular surgical procedures. *Surg Gynecol Obstet.* 1971;133:59–65.
7. Shealy CN, Mortimer JT, Reswick JB. Electrical inhibition of pain by stimulation of the dorsal columns: preliminary clinical report. *Anesth Analg.* 1967;46(3):489–91.
8. Melzack R, Wall P. Pain Mechanisms: A New Theory. *Science.* 1965;150(3699):971–9.
9. Melzack R, Wall P. On the nature of cutaneous sensory mechanisms. *Brain.* 1962;85(2):331-56.
10. Melzack R. Pain: Past, present and future. *Canadian J of Experimental Psychology.* 1993;47(4):615–29.
11. Descartes R, Hall TS. *Treatise of Man.* Cambridge: Harvard University Press; 1972.
12. Moayedi M, Davis KD. Theories of pain: from specificity to gate control. *J Neurophysiol.* 2013;109:5-12.
13. Melzack R, Jones C. *The Day Tuk Became a Hunter and other Eskimo Stories.* 1st ed. New York: Mead; 1967.
14. Cohen L. An anesthetist of a different order. *Canadian Medical Association Journal.* 1999;160:160.
15. Cousins MJ. Oral History Interview with Michael J. Cousins, John C. Liebeskind History of Pain Collection. 19 October 1997 [Interviewed by: Meldrum ML].
16. Loeser JD. In Memoriam: John J. Bonica. *Pain.* 1994;59(1).
17. Mazze RI, Trudell JR, Cousins MJ. Methoxyflurane metabolism and renal dysfunction: clinical correlation in man. *Anesthesiology.* 1971;35:247-52.
18. Cousins MJ, Mazze RI. Methoxyflurane nephrotoxicity: a study of dose response in man. *JAMA.* 1973;225(13):1611–6.

19. Jones L. *First Steps. The early years of IASP. 1973-1984*. Seattle: IASP Press; 2010.
20. Loeser JD. Personal interview. 28 September 2019 [Interviewed by: Kelly-Davies G].
21. Foley K. Personal interview. 26 September 2019 [Interviewed by: Kelly-Davies G].
22. Russo M. *The Michael J Cousins Lifetime Achievement Award* International Neuromodulation Society Annual Scientific Meeting; Sydney May 2019.
23. Cousins MJ. *Doctorate of Medicine Thesis: Anaesthetic toxicity: Metabolism and nephrotoxicity of fluorinated inhalation anaesthetics*. University of Sydney; 1975.
24. Haynes J. Adelaide apocalypse: South Australia in the 70s took the cake for fake news. *The Guardian*. 22 December 2016. Available from: https://www.theguardian.com/australia-news/2016/dec/22/adelaide-apocalypse-south-australia-in-the-70s-took-the-cake-for-fake-news. Accessed 5 April 2020.
25. Dunstan D. *ALP policy speech: The Radical Dream. Social Reform in South Australia*. State Library of South Australia 1970.
26. Harris R. Personal interview. 30 August 2019 [Interviewed by: Kelly-Davies G].
27. Mather LE. Personal interview. 16 April 2019 [Interviewed by: Kelly-Davies G].
28. SA Team Smashes Pain Barrier. *The News*. 8 November 1978
29. Basbaum A. Personal interview. 19 December 2019 [Interviewed by: Kelly-Davies G].
30. Godden J. *Australian Pain Society: The First 35 Years*. North Sydney: Australian Pain Society; 2015.
31. Rounsefell B. Personal interview. 11 November 2019 [Interviewed by: Kelly-Davies G].
32. Fink BR. History of Local Anesthesia. In: Cousins MJ, Bridenbaugh P, editors. *Neural Blockade in Clinical Anaesthesia and Management of Pain*. Philadelphia: J. B. Lippincott Co.; 1980. p. 6–12.
33. Doughty A. Walter Stoeckel (1871-1961). A pioneer of regional analgesia in obstetrics. *Anaesthesia*. 1990;45:468-71.
34. Stoeckel W. Über sakrale anästhesie. *Zentralblatt für Gynäkologie*.1909;33:1–15.
35. Yasch T. Personal interview. 25 September 2019 [Interviewed by: Kelly-Davies G].
36. Cousins MJ, Mather LE, Glynn CJ, Wilson, P.R., Graham JR. Selective Spinal Anaesthesia. *The Lancet*. 1979;1(8126):11141–2.
37. Glynn CJ, Mather LE, Cousins MJ, Wilson PR, Graham JR. Spinal narcotics and respiratory depression. *The Lancet*. 1979;2(8138):356–7

38. Cousins MJ, Bridenbaugh PO, editors. *Neural Blockade in Clinical Anesthesia and Management of Pain* 1st ed. Philadelphia: J. B. Lippincott Company; 1980.
39. Carr DB. Personal interview. 18 July 2019 [Interviewed by: Kelly-Davies G].
40. Basbaum A. *Michael J. Cousins Doctor of Science Thesis, Examiner's report*. University of California, San Francisco; 2006.
41. Frankl VE. *Man's Search for Meaning*. Boston: Beacon Press; 1946.
42. Cousins G. Personal interview. 25 September 2019 [Interviewed by: Kelly-Davies G].
43. Cousins MJ, Mather LE. Intrathecal and epidural administration of opioids. *Anesthesiology*. 1984;61:276–309.
44. Shipton T. Honouring a giant in the field of pain medicine. A pain medicine perspective. *ANZCA Bulletin*. December 2016.
45. Cherry DA. Drug delivery systems for epidural administration of opioids. *Acta Anaesthesiol Scand Suppl*. 1987;31(Supplementum 85):54–9.
46. Loeser JD. Wilbert E. Fordyce, Ph.D. 1923–2009. *Pain*. 2010;148:1–2.
47. Cornwall J. *After Work, After Play, After All: A Political Memoir* Adelaide: Bookpod; 8 September 2017.
48. Cherry DA, Gourlav GK, McLachlan M, Cousins MJ. Diagnostic epidural opioid blockade in chronic pain. *Pain*. 1984;21:143-52.
49. Boylen L. Clinic breaks the pain barrier. *The Weekend Australian*. 17–18 August 1985.
50. Cherry DA, Gourlay GK, McLachlan M, Cousins MJ. Diagnostic epidural opioid blockade in chronic pain. *Pain*. 1985;21:143-52.
51. Cherry DA, Gourlay GK, Cousins MJ, Gannon BJ. A technique for the insertion of an implantable portal system for the long-term administration of opioids in the treatment of cancer pain. *Anaesth Intensive Care*. 1985;13:145–52.
52. Cousins MJ. Letter to Holland R. 6 February 1986.
53. Gross P. *The economic costs of chronic pain in Australia*. Eighth Annual Scientific Meeting of the Australian Pain Society; Melbourne 5–7 February 1986.
54. Melzack R. IASP President's Message. *IASP Newsletter*. August 1987.
55. Cousins MJ. Incoming IASP President's Message. *IASP Newsletter*. August 1987.
56. NHMRC. *Management of Severe Pain*: Australian Government Publishing Service; 1988.
57. Cousins MJ. JJ Bonica Lecture: Acute pain and the injury response: immediate and prolonged effects. *Reg Anesth Pain Medicine*. 1989;14:162–78.
58. Cousins MJ, Mather LE. Relief of postoperative pain: advances awaiting application. *MJA*. 1989;150:354–6.

59. Cousins MJ, Knights KM, Gourlay GK, Hall PD, Lunam CA, O'Brien P. A randomised prospective study of the metabolism and hepatotoxicity of halothane in man. *Anesth Analg.* 1987;66:299–308.
60. Cousins MJ, Loeser J. *Studies of epidemiology of chronic pain.* Fulbright Commission; 1989.
61. Loeser JD, editor *Desirable characteristics for pain treatment facilities: report of the IASP Taskforce.* Sixth World Congress on Pain; 1990; Adelaide: IASP.
62. IASP Task Force. *Desirable Characteristics for Pain Treatment Facilities* Boston: IASP; 1990. Available from: https://www.iasp-pain.org/Education/Content.aspx?ItemNumber=1471, accessed 8 March 2021.
63. Loeser JD, Van Konkelenberg R, Volinn E, Cousins MJ. Small area analysis of lumbar spine surgery in South Australia. *Aust NZ J Surg.* 1993;63:14–9.
64. Cousins C. Personal interview. 25 May 2020 [Interviewed by: Kelly-Davies G].
65. Spring S. Personal interview. 24 April 2020 [Interviewed by: Kelly-Davies G].
66. Spring S. In: Cousins MJ, editor. NSW Northern Area Health Service; 9 May 1990.
67. Sarzin A. First Australian Chair of Anaesthesia and Pain Management. *Radius.* 1991:2.
68. Cousins J. Personal interview. 6 May 2020 [Interviewed by:Kelly-Davies G].
69. Cousins MJ, Gallagher RM. *Fast Facts: Chronic and Cancer Pain* 4th ed. Oxford: Health Press Limited; 2017 June 2017.
70. Nock P. Personal interview. 25 May 2020 [Interviewed by: Kelly-Davies G].
71. Molloy A. Personal interview. 3 October 2019 [Interviewed by: Kelly-Davies G].
72. Russo M. Personal interview. 17 January 2021 [Interviewed by: Kelly-Davies G].
73. Siddall PJ. Personal interview. 1 August 2019 [Interviewed by: Kelly-Davies G.].
74. Siddall PJ, Taylor DA, Cousins MJ. Classification of pain following spinal cord injury. *Spinal Cord.* 1997;35:69–75.
75. Siddall PJ, Xu CL, Cousins MJ. Allodynia following traumatic spinal cord injury in the rat. *NeuroReport.* 1995;6:1241–4.
76. Siddall PJ, Xu CL, Keay KA, Cousins MJ. Increased fos expression in dorsal horn of spinal cord in rats displaying allodynia following spinal cord injury. *Proc Aust Neuroscience Soc.* 1996;7:233.
77. Siddall PJ, Molloy AR, Walker S, Mather LE, Rutkowski SB, Cousins MJ. The efficacy of intrathecal morphine and clonidine in the treatment of pain after spinal cord injury. *Anesth Analg.* 2000;91(6):1493–98.

78. Siddall PJ, Cousins MJ, Otte A, Griesing T, Chambers R, Murphy TK. Pregabalin in central neuropathic pain associated with spinal cord injury: a placebo-controlled trial. *Neurology.* 2006;67:1792–800.
79. Siddall PJ, McClelland JM, Rutkowski SP, Cousins MJ. A longitudinal study of the prevalence and characteristics of pain in the first five years following spinal cord injury. *Pain.* 2002;103:249–57.
80. Keith Cousins is inducted into AdNews Hall of Fame. *AdNews.* 27 November 2012.
81. Moskowitz MH, Golden MD. *Neuroplastic Transformation. Your Brain on Pain Workbook* USA: Neuroplastic Partners; 2013.
82. M Robyn. Personal interview. 25 May 2020 [Interviewed by: Kelly-Davies G.].
83. Grewal J. Personal interview. 24 May 2020 [Interviewed by: Kelly-Davies G.].
84. Nicholas M. Personal interview. 25 September 2019 [Interviewed by: Kelly-Davies G].
85. Molloy AR. Personal interview. 3 October 2019 [Interviewed by: Kelly-Davies G].
86. Liu S. Email interview. 19 May 2020 [Interviewed by: Kelly-Davies G].
87. Frend C. Personal interview. 11 December 2019 [Interviewed by: Kelly-Davies G].
88. AIHW. *Australia's Health 2018.* Canberra; 20 June 2018.
89. Votrubec M. Personal interview. 30 April 2019 [Interviewed by: Kelly-Davies G].
90. Glare P. Personal interview. 17 April 2019 [Interviewed by: Kelly-Davies G].
91. Cousins MJ, Power I, Smith G. Pain – A Persistent Problem. Gaston Labat Lecture. *Reg Anesth Pain Medicine.* 2000;25:6–21.
92. Johnston H. Personal interview. 18 August 2019 [Interviewed by: Kelly-Davies G].
93. Cousins MJ. Pain: The Past, Present and Future of Anesthesiology? The E.A. Rovenstine Memorial Lecture. *Anesthesiology.*1999;91:538–51.
94. Cousins MJ. Phase Two - Opening Report Pain Management and Research Centre *Centre for Anaesthesia and Pain Research Newsletter.* March 1997.
95. Shipton EA, Moore B, Cousins MJ, Atkinson L. Commentary. The Faculty of Pain Medicine of the Australian and New Zealand College of Anaesthetists – History and Strategic Plan. *Pain Medicine.* 2014;15.
96. Cousins MJ. Faculty of Pain Medicine Dean's Message. *ANZCA Bulletin.* 2002;12(2).
97. Jones MR, Viswanath O, Peck J, Kaye AD, Gill JS, Simopoulos TT. A Brief History of the Opioid Epidemic and Strategies for Pain Medicine. *Pain Ther.* 2018;7(1):13-21.

98. AIHW. *Opioid harm in Australia: and comparisons between Australia and Canada.* Canberra: Australian Government; 9 November 2018.
99. Bell J. Australian trends in opioid prescribing for chronic non-cancer pain, 1986–1996. *MJA.* 1997;167:30–4.
100. Molloy AR, Nicholas MJ, Cousins MJ. Role of opioids in chronic non-cancer pain. *MJA.* 1997;167:9–10.
101. Royal North Shore Hospital. *Centre for Anaesthesia and Pain Management Research submission* NHMRC Centres of Clinical Excellence in Hospital-based Research: 1998.
102. Geoffrey Kaye Museum. *Pain and Progress. The formation and development of the Faculty of Pain Medicine* Melbourne: ANZCA; 2014. Available from: https://www.geoffreykayemuseum.org.au/faculty-of-pain-medicine-history/, accessed 4 November 2019.
103. Cousins MJ. Faculty of Pain Medicine Dean's Message. *ANZCA Bulletin.* 1999;8(1).
104. Goucke R. Personal interview. 23 October 2019 [Interviewed by: Kelly-Davies G].
105. Royal College of Anaesthetists. *Faculty of Pain Medicine* London: Royal College of Anaesthetists. Available from: https://www.fpm.ac.uk/about-faculty, accessed 8 March 2021.
106. Arnold C. Personal interview. 9 October 2019 [Interviewed by: Kelly-Davies G].
107. McIntyre P. Personal interview. 3 October 2019 [Interviewed by: Kelly-Davies G].
108. NHMRC. *Acute Pain Management: Scientific Evidence.* NHMRC; 1999.
109. Parnell S. The relief of severe pain was a basic human right. *Courier Mail.* 1999 15 July 1999.
110. Gray D. The Cost Of Pain Hurts The Nation's Economy. *The Age* 13 July 1999.
111. Pain relief cost effective and a basic human right *Australian Associated Press*; 12 July 1999.
112. Walker S. Personal interview. 27 August 2019 [Interviewed by: Kelly-Davies G].
113. Vaughan C. Personal interview. 20 August 2019 [Interviewed by: Kelly-Davies G].
114. Kipling R, Karlin D. *Rudyard Kipling* Oxford: Oxford University Press; 1999.
115. Davidson B. Personal interview. 23 July 2019 [Interviewed by: Kelly-Davies G].
116. Brooker C. Personal interview. 13 August 2019 [Interviewed by: Kelly-Davies G].

117. Cousins MJ. Faculty of Pain Medicine Dean's Message. *ANZCA Bulletin.* 2000;9(3).
118. Blyth F, March L, Brnabic AJM, Jorm LR, Williamson M, Cousins M. Chronic pain in Australia: a prevalence study. *Pain.* 2001;89:127–34.
119. Cousins MJ. Faculty of Pain Medicine Dean's Message. *ANZCA Bulletin.* 2000;9(1).
120. Cousins MJ. Faculty of Pain Medicine Dean's Message. *ANZCA Bulletin.* 2000;9(2).
121. Cousins MJ. Faculty of Pain Medicine Dean's Message. *ANZCA Bulletin.* 2000;9(4).
122. Cousins MJ. Faculty of Pain Medicine Dean's Message. *ANZCA Bulletin.* 2002;11(1).
123. Siddall PJ, Cousins MJ. Persistent pain as a disease entity: implications for clinical management. *Anesth Analg.* 2004;99:510–20.
124. Cousins MJ. *In response to 'Is chronic pain a disease in its own right?':* Body In Mind; 2011. Available from: https://bodyinmind.org/prof-cousins-response-is-chronic-pain-a-disease/, accessed 17 August 2020.
125. Lau B. Personal interview. 25 August 2019 [Interviewed by: Kelly-Davies G].
126. Cohen M. Personal interview. 1 October 2019 [Interviewed by: Kelly-Davies G].
127. Blyth F, March L, Cousins M. Chronic Pain-Related Disability and Use of Analgesia and Health Services in a Sydney Community. *MJA.* 2003; 179(2):84–7.
128. Blyth F, March L, Nicholas M, Cousins M. Self-Management of Chronic Pain: A Population-Based Study. *Pain.* 2005;11(3):285–92.
129. Van Leeuwen MT, Blyth FM, March LM, Nicholas MK, Cousins MJ. Chronic pain and reduced work effectiveness: the hidden cost to Australian employers. *Eur J Pain.* 2006;10(2):161–6.
130. Access Economics. *The High Price of Pain. The Economic Impact of Persistent Pain in Australia.* November 2007.
131. McLean T. Pain comes with $34 billion price tag. *Australian Associated Press* 19 November 2007.
132. Blyth F. Personal interview. 20 December 2019 [Interviewed by: Kelly-Davies G].
133. Lau B. *Change or Die: The Future of Multidisciplinary Pain Centers*: The University of Sydney; 2008.
134. RNS department head says he's at his wit's end: *Australian Associated Press*, 14 March 2008.
135. Garling P. *Final Report of the Special Commission of Inquiry: Acute Care in NSW Public Hospitals.* 27 November 2008.

136. Brydon L. Personal interview. 12 April 2019 [Interviewed by: Kelly-Davies G].
137. Sparkes D. Taking research to Europe. *The Observer (Gladstone)*. 20 May 2011.
138. Brydon L. Personal interview. 8 April 2019 [Interviewed by: Kelly-Davies G].
139. Skilton N. Taking pains. *Australian Doctor.* 9 September 2011.
140. Parker J. Personal interview. 17 September 2019 [Interviewed by: Kelly-Davies G].
141. Fry R. Personal communication. 19 September 2019 [Interviewed by: Kelly-Davies G].
142. Pierik P. Management of chronic pain 'inadequate'. AAP Bulletins [Internet]. *Australian Associated Press*; 2009.
143. Calls for a new way of dealing with pain: *Australian Broadcasting Corporation* 19 October 2009.
144. Institute of Medicine. *National Pain Strategy Report. A Comprehensive Population Health-Level Strategy for Pain.* Washington: National Institutes of Health 2011.
145. Cousins MJ. *Michael Cousins speech notes.* National Pain Summit; Canberra 11 March 2010.
146. Cousins MJ. Chronic pain summit opens, *The World Today.* 11 March 2010 [Interviewed by: Hall E].
147. Cousins MJ. Painful reality – patients let down, *7.30 Report.* 11 March 2010 [Interviewed by: O'Brien K].
148. Atkinson L. Personal interview. 1 October 2019 [Interviewed by: Kelly-Davies G].
149. Wrigley P. Personal interview. 20 August 2019 [Interviewed by: Kelly-Davies G].
150. IASP. *Declaration of Montreal.* Boston: IASP; 3 September 2010.
151. Gallagher R. Personal interview. 19 September 2019 [Interviewed by: Kelly-Davies G].
152. Cousins MJ, Lynch M. The Declaration of Montreal: Access to pain management is a fundamental human right. *Pain.* 2011;152:2673–4.
153. Sukel K. A 10-Year Anniversary: Reflecting on the Declaration of Montreal, IASP. *Pain Research Forum.* 1 August 2020.
154. National Institute on Drug Abuse. *Opioid Overdose Crisis.* Washington: National Institutes of Health; 2021.
155. Roxburgh A, Dobbins T, Degenhardt L, Peacock A. *Opioid, amphetamine, and cocaine-induced deaths in Australia.* National Drug and Alcohol Research Centre, UNSW 2018.
156. Skinner J. Personal interview. 24 April 2019 [Interviewed by: Kelly-Davies G].
157. Pain to be a priority. *Pain Pals.* September 2011.

158. State Government to set up pain taskforce. *St George & Sutherland Shire Leader.* 10 May 2011.
159. Johnson J. Personal interview. 19 April 2019 [Interviewed by: Kelly-Davies G].
160. *NSW leads national bid to see chronic pain recognised as a disease* [press release]. Sydney: NSW Health Minister. 14 June 2013.
161. Bonnie R. Pain Management and Opioid Regulation: Continuing Public Health Challenges. *AJPH.* 2019;109(1):31–4.
162. Hotz P. Personal interview. 21 May 2020 [Interviewed by: Kelly-Davies G].
163. *An overhaul for pain management in NSW* [press release]. Sydney: NSW Health Minister. 18 July 2012.
164. Chang C. Dedicated to research. *North Shore Times.* 14 February 2014.
165. The Governor-General of the Commonwealth of Australia. *Australia Day 2014 Honours List* Canberra: Australian Government; 26 January 2014. Available from: https://www.gg.gov.au/australia-day-2014-honours-list, accessed 26 February 2021.
166. Schug S. Personal interview. 2019 [Interviewed by: Kelly-Davies G].
167. Faculty of Pain Medicine email correspondence. February 2021.
168. RACGP. *General Practice: Health of the Nation 2020.* East Melbourne, Vic: RACGP; 2020.
169. *RNSH Renamed in Honour of Professor Michael Cousins* [press release]. NSW Health Minister 11 February 2014.
170. Cousins MJ. *Michael Cousins speech notes* Renaming event Michael J Cousins Centre for Pain Management; Royal North Shore Hospital 11 February 2014.
171. Skinner J. *Health Minister Speech Notes* Renaming ceremony Michael J Cousins Centre for Pain Management; Royal North Shore Hospital 11 February 2014.
172. Kerin L. *Patient fitted with world-first spinal cord stimulator to treat chronic pain at Royal North Shore Hospital* Sydney: Australian Broadcasting Corporation; 15 October 2015. Available from: https://www.abc.net.au/news/2015-10-15/patient-fitted-with-spinal-cord-stimulator-to-treat-chronic-pain/6856792, accessed 3 January 2020.
173. Russo M. *Long-Term Results from the Avalon Study: Feedback SCS Using Evoked Compound Action Potentials (Closed-Loop SCS).* International Neuromodulation Society 14th World Congress. Sydney 25–30 May 2019.
174. Russo M, Brooker C, Cousins MJ, Taylor N, Boesel T, Sullivan R, et al. Sustained Long-Term Outcomes With Closed-Loop Spinal Cord Stimulation: 12-Month Results of the Prospective, Multicenter, Open-Label Avalon Study. *Neurosurgery.* 2020;87(4):485–95.
175. Brooker C. *A festschrift presentation in honour of Michael J. Cousins AO.* Festchrift presentation; Kolling Institute, Royal North Shore Hospital 19 May 2016.

176. Parker J. *Festschrift. Professor Michael J. Cousins AO* 19 May 2016.
177. Cousins MJ. *Michael Cousins speech notes* Festschrift presentation in honour of Michael J Cousins AO, Royal North Shore Hospital 19 May 2016.
178. *Saluda Medical Announces Clinical Study Results for Evoke® ECAP-Controlled, Closed-Loop SCS System for the Treatment of Chronic Pain* [press release]. Sydney: PR Newswire 3 June 2019.
179. Russo M, Cousins MJ, Brooker C, Taylor N, Boesel T, Sullivan R, et al. Effective Relief of Pain and Associated Symptoms With Closed-Loop Spinal Cord Stimulation System: Preliminary Results of the Avalon Study. *Neuromodulation.* 2018;21(1):38–47.
180. *Painaustralia welcomes new CEO* [press release]. Canberra: Painaustralia 29 May 2017.
181. *At last – A national plan for better pain management* [press release]. Canberra: Painaustralia 17 June 2019.
182. *$6.8 million to improve understanding of pain* [press release]. Canberra: Federal Health Minister 4 April 2019.
183. Bennett C. Personal interview. 19 February 2020 [Interviewed by: Kelly-Davies G].
184. Australian Chronic Pain Sufferers Facebook Group. Facebook; accessed 12 October 2020.
185. NSW Agency for Clinical Innovation. *Pain Management Network Website* Sydney: NSW Government; 2012. Available from: https://www.aci.health.nsw.gov.au/chronic-pain. accessed 5 January 2020.
186. Australian Pain Management Association Website. *Australian Pain Management Association* 2018. Available from: https://www.painmanagement.org.au/, accessed 17 August 2020.
187. Painaustralia. *Patient support groups around Australia* Canberra: Painaustralia; 2020. Available from: https://www.painaustralia.org.au/find-support/care-in-community-1/painaustralia-support-groups-help-lines, accessed 8 March 2021.
188. Chronic Pain Australia Website. *Chronic Pain Australia.* Available from: https://chronicpainaustralia.org.au/index.php, accessed 17 August 2020.
189. *Professor Michael Cousins AM. Nomination for Australian of the Year* [press release]. Canberra: Painaustralia 2012.
190. European Pain Federation. *Societal Impact of Pain Platform* Brussels. Available from: https://www.sip-platform.eu/en, accessed 9 March 2021.
191. Committee on Advancing Pain Research Care and Education. *Relieving Pain in America: A Blueprint for Transforming Prevention, Care, Education, and Research.* Washington D.C.: Institute of Medicine.

192. United States Interagency Pain Research Coordinating Committee. *National Pain Strategy*. Washington D.C.: National Institute of Health; 2016.
193. NSW Government. *NSW Pain Management Plan 2012–2016 NSW Government Response to the Pain Management Taskforce Report* May 2012.
194. National Academy of Sciences. *Relieving Pain in America, a Blueprint for Transforming Prevention, Care, Education and Research*. Washington D.C.: US Institute of Medicine.
195. Treede RD, Rief W, Barke A. Chronic pain as a symptom or a disease: the IASP classification of chronic pain for the International Classification of Diseases. *Pain.* January 2019;160(1):19–27.
196. World Health Organization. *International Classification of Diseases 11th Edition* 2020. Available from: https://icd.who.int/en, accessed 9 August 2020.

Book reviews can make or break a book. If you liked what you read today, please do consider posting an online review on Goodreads or your favourite forum.

Breaking Through the Pain Barrier is available
at www.hawkeyebooks.com.au
and all good bookstores and libraries.

Proudly supported by

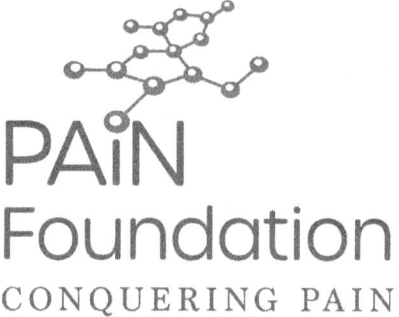

www.ingramcontent.com/pod-product-compliance
Lightning Source LLC
Chambersburg PA
CBHW071959290426
44109CB00018B/2066